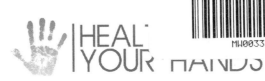

An Essential Guide for
Scoliosis and a Healthy Pregnancy

About Dr Kevin Lau

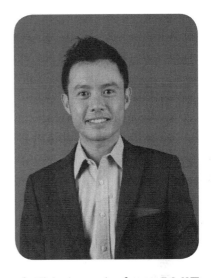

Dr Kevin Lau is the founder of Health In Your Hands, a series of tools for Scoliosis prevention and treatment. The set includes his book Your Plan for Natural Scoliosis Prevention and Treatment (available in English, Spanish, Chinese, Japanese, Korean, Italian, French and German), a companion Scoliosis Exercises for Prevention and Correction DVD, and the innovative new mobile application ScolioTrack for iPhone, iPad and Android devices.

Dr Kevin Lau is a graduate in Doctor of Chiropractic from RMIT University in Melbourne Australia and Masters in Holistic Nutrition. Dr Kevin Lau is a member of International Society On Scoliosis Orthopedic and Rehabilitation Treatment (SOSORT), the leading international society on conservative treatment of spinal deformities and the American Chiropractic Association (ACA) the largest professional association in the United States.

He was the first in Singapore to provide a non-surgical treatment for scoliosis in Singapore 2005 first by studying the Schroth Method of Exercises and then working in a clinic which implemented Clear Institute Methods. During this time he has been devoted to developing, practicing, and teaching others about non-surgical solutions for scoliosis. He has completed 3 theses "The role of calcium and vitamin D in the prevention of low bone density and Adolescent Idiopathic Scoliosis (AIS) in prepubertal women." With his research into spinal conditions he is the published author of Your Plan for Natural Scoliosis Prevention and Treatment which has been translated to Chinese, Japanese, Spanish, French and German. Dr. Lau combines a university education and a lifetime of practicing natural and preventive medicine to provide a unique approach to health care.

He made it his aim in life to explore & share the truths about nutrition, diseases and healing and educate patients from all walks of life around the world. He is a recipient of the Best Health-care Provider Award by the Straits Time, the leading newspaper publication in Singapore and featured on TV, PrimeTime Channel News Asia.

To find out more about who Dr Kevin Lau is, please visit his website, www.HIYH.info.

Chat with him on Facebook, Twitter, Google+ or blog. He would love to hear from you!

www.facebook.com/healthinyourhands

www.twitter.com/drkevinlau

www.gplus.to/drkevinlau

www.drkevinlau.blogspot.com

Dr. Kevin Lau's Mission Statement

The true cure for scoliosis lies in the eradication of its root cause. I, hereby reinforce my commitment to the research to unravel the factors that cause scoliosis. The current research is limited to the analysis of bracing and surgical techniques which only treat the symptoms and impact of the disorder. The research to identify and treat the core cause of scoliosis still offers a vast scope.

Towards this end, I promise to dedicate a portion of proceeds of my books to the research focused on understanding the root cause of scoliosis, which will help us protect our future generations from this widespread spinal deformity.

FOREWORD

In today's Information Age, the internet can be a confusing and unreliable resource for those seeking answers to their unique medical conditions. It can be challenging to sift through this information and determine what is reliable or medically authoritative. Reading this book will provide the much-awaited answers to queries regarding two of the most important aspects of pregnancy in scoliosis – Nutrition & Exercise.

I feel humbled to have been offered the opportunity to prepare the foreword for such an important book. Dr. Kevin Lau's endeavour to author a book on pregnancy and scoliosis is a commendable undertaking, as the topic is one that perplexes many people indeed. Who could be better able to share his expert knowledge and ability to understand the complexities of getting pregnant with scoliosis than an experienced chiropractor? Dr. Kevin Lau is a graduate in Doctor of Chiropractic from RMIT University, Melbourne (Australia) and holds a Masters in Holistic Nutrition. He is also a member of the International Society on Scoliosis Orthopaedic and Rehabilitation Treatment (SOSORT).

This is a wonderful source of information for scoliotic patients who wish to enjoy the process of their pregnancy while taking care of their baby in the healthiest possible manner. I recommend this book for anybody who wants to understand how scoliosis may affect their pregnancy and what steps can be taken in order to safeguard their health.

Dr. Siddhant Kapoor, M.B.B.S, D.N.B.
Orthopaedic Surgeon

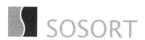

SOSORT

INTERNATIONAL *SOCIETY* ON *SCOLIOSIS* *ORTHOPAEDIC* AND *REHABILITATION* *TREATMENT*

In recognition of his contributions to the care and conservative treatment of scoliosis

Kevin LAU, DC

Singapore, Singapore

is hereby declared
Associate *Member of* **SOSORT** *in 2012*

Stefano Negrini, MD, Italy
President

Patrick Knott, PhD, PA-C
General Secretary

ACA American Chiropractic Association

THE AMERICAN CHIROPRACTIC ASSOCIATION IS PLEASED TO GRANT THIS CERTIFICATE OF MEMBERSHIP TO

Kevin Lau, D.C.

I HEREBY CERTIFY THAT THIS DOCTOR OF CHIROPRACTIC IS A MEMBER OF THE AMERICAN CHIROPRACTIC ASSOCIATION, WHICH SUPPORTS PATIENTS' RIGHTS AND PATIENT TREATMENT REIMBURSEMENT, AND HAS PLEDGED TO ABIDE BY THE ACA CODE OF ETHICS, WHICH IS BASED UPON THE FUNDAMENTAL PRINCIPLE THAT THE PARAMOUNT PURPOSE OF THE CHIROPRACTOR'S PROFESSIONAL SERVICES SHALL BE TO BENEFIT THE PATIENT.

Keith S. Overland, DC
President

April 17, 2012
Date

ACA's PURPOSE
To provide leadership in health care and a positive vision for the chiropractic profession and its natural approach to health and wellness

ACA's MISSION
To preserve, protect, improve and promote the chiropractic profession and the services of Doctors of Chiropractic for the benefit of patients they serve

ACA's VISION
To transform health care from a focus on disease to a focus on wellness

An Essential Guide for
Scoliosis and a Healthy Pregnancy

Month-by-month, everything you need to know about taking care of your spine and baby.

By Dr. Kevin Lau D.C.
Foreword by Dr. Siddhant Kapoor M.D.

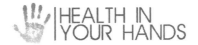

Dr. Kevin Lau
302 Orchard Road #06-03,
Tong Building (Rolex Centre),
Singapore 238862.

For more information about the companion Exercise DVD, Audiobook and ScolioTrack App for iPhone, Android or iPad visit:

www.HIYH.info
www.ScolioTrack.com

Printed in the United States of America

ISBN: 9810718101
EAN-13: 9789810718107

Disclaimer

The information contained in this book is for educational purposes only. It is not intended to be used to diagnose or treat any disease, and is not a substitute or a prescription for proper medical advice, intervention, or treatment. Any consequences resulting from the application of this information will be the sole responsibility of the reader. Neither the authors nor the publishers will be liable for any damages caused, or alleged to be caused, by the application of the information in this book. Individuals with a known or suspected health condition are strongly encouraged to seek advice of a licensed healthcare professional before implementing any of the protocols in this book.

Dedication

This book is dedicated to my family and patients, whose love, support, and inspiration helped me to piece together a better understanding of the workings of the spine and optimal health.

Aknowledgement

MicroArts (Graphic Designer, Pakistan) — For designing the layout of the entire book and various inputs into making the book easier to read and artistic direction.

Nemanja Stankovic (Illustrator, Serbia) — Who drew all the amazing illustrations in the book and the beautiful image for the book cover.

Dr. Siddhant Kapoor (Editor, Orthopaedic Doctor) — For his pervasive commitment to quality and keeping me abreast with the latest medical research.

Bebe Battsetseg (Model, Mongolia) — Who learned and demonstrated all the exercises in the book to perfection.

Jericho Soh Chee Loon (Photographer, Singapore) - For all the professionally taken photos.

TABLE OF CONTENTS

Pregnancy and Scoliosis
An Introduction

If you are intrigued enough to read this book, I may assume that you are already aware of what scoliosis is and are getting worried about its effect on your pregnancy. While you may have gathered some information about scoliosis, the subject is still under a lot of research and consideration among medical professionals.

This is mainly due to the fact that researchers are still not successful in unraveling the reasons and factors that cause scoliosis. Most conventional physicians also claim that there is no cure for scoliosis and that it can only be managed with bracing and surgery.

On the other hand, you may also come across physicians who are of the opinion that the surgical correction of scoliosis is merely a symptomatic treatment to correct the curve. There have been cases mentioned in the literature where the symptoms and deformity due to scoliosis has returned back to its original curve in less than five years after the surgery.

There are various theories, still under discussion, regarding factors that cause scoliosis. While there is still no unanimity about the specific cause and treatment, there is an empirical data that shows that a good holistic diet specifically-targeted exercises and healthy living can help scoliosis patients lead an extremely happy and comfortable life.

Pregnancy is a tough time for all women, regardless of whether you have scoliosis or not. While there are a large number of symptoms, starting from the first trimester to the time of delivery, there is no way to know the specific symptoms that will manifest themselves in your pregnancy. While some suffer with a sensation of nausea during the first few months of pregnancy, others feel no discomfort at all. There are still others who may experience acid reflux throughout the nine months of pregnancy.

While there are no set patterns when it comes to the kind of pregnancy that you will experience, there are some guidelines that may be helpful in making it a wonderful experience. Given that you carry an extra load inside you at least during the last trimester, the amount of weight and pressure that it puts on your spine is immense. Even expecting mothers without scoliosis curves are advised against lifting heavy weights or doing exercises that can damage the spine for a lifetime.

Expecting mothers with scoliosis need to be aware of some specific aspects. This is because while they need to be careful about all the regular aspects of pregnancy, they need to do so with an extra care due to their scoliosis. When expecting mothers with scoliosis are aware of the complications that their condition may cause, they can prepare themselves to prevent the situation from getting worse.

It will be a great relief for you to know that suffering from scoliosis during pregnancy neither rules out a normal delivery nor does it mean that you cannot have a healthy baby. It does not always lead to complications during pregnancy either. Have heart and read on to know what you need to do in order to ensure that your curved back does not alter your pregnancy.

CHAPTER 1

WHAT IS SCOLIOSIS?

Complete knowledge about scoliosis will help you understand your situation in the best possible way. This is why it is important that you comprehend all aspects of scoliosis so that you are able to combat the condition in an aware and informed manner. It may not always be practical enough to pick up the phone and speak to your health care advisor or it may not be feasible for you to make a trip to the doctor every other day to get your query answered. Yet questions about your pregnancy and the effect that scoliosis has on it may arise in your curious mind at every stage of your pregnancy.

It is likely that you have specific symptoms at each stage of pregnancy that may make you wonder whether they are caused due to scoliosis. The pain in your back may be a normal part of pregnancy or may be caused by your scoliosis. You may be curious whether the acid reflux that you are facing is a part of the process of pregnancy and whether you can change something in your diet to avoid this or not. To be able to answer many of these questions on your own and be self-assured, you need to understand what scoliosis is, the symptoms that may appear during each stage of your pregnancy, the manner in which each of these symptoms may be aggravated during pregnancy, the factors that cause the condition and the manner in which it can affect your child.

It is also important that you check out all the possible treatment options that are available for scoliosis and understand the fact that you are not alone. There are many women who get pregnant while suffering from scoliosis. The scoliosis progresses at a higher rate in

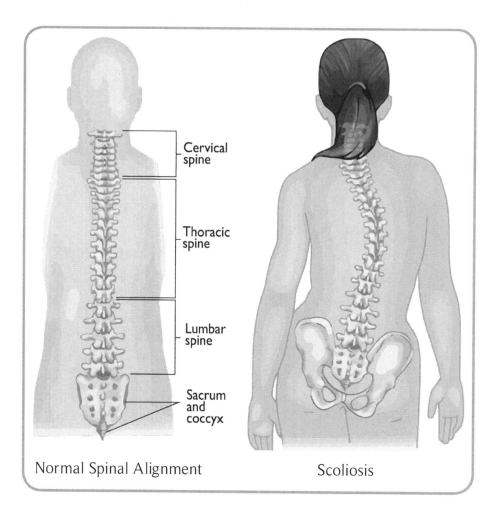

Cervical spine	
Thoracic spine	
Lumbar spine	
Sacrum and coccyx	

Normal Spinal Alignment   Scoliosis

women than in men but a large number of these women are also able to give normal birth to their babies.

Without increasing your inquisitiveness any further let us begin the process of educating ourselves about the various aspects of scoliosis.

Scoliosis is a medical condition that affects about 3-5 out of 1000 people worldwide and it affects more than 7 million people in the United States. The ironic part is that there are a large number of people who suffer from this condition without it ever being detected. This is because many physicians may miss mild symptoms of scoliosis. Sometimes they may get ignored completely even on being detected because the person is too old for invasive treatments which could be risky.

Since there is no unanimous understanding of the factors that cause the condition or any treatment that can be provided to cure those who have mild scoliosis, most doctors just choose to avoid mentioning it to the patient. Later in this book, you will find how you could ask a friend for help or check at home whether you have any cause for concern and whether you should visit a physician to confirm your possibility of having scoliosis at all.

Scoliosis has a Greek origin from the word 'skolios' that means crooked. This is because scoliosis is a condition in which the spine is curved in an abnormal manner. When you look at a normal spine from the rear it appears straight. The frontal view of the spine should be a straight line in people who do not have a scoliosis curve. Among those who have a scoliosis condition, the spine is curved.

The location where the curve appears may vary in different women. In some cases there is a single curve, while in others there may be multiple curves at different locations along the spine. In most cases, the shape of the spine may appear 'S' shaped or 'C' shaped.

In most people, scoliosis appears between 10 and 15 years of age. The majority of the cases diagnosed is from this age group. The condition is higher among females and the ratio of affection of females to males is 3.6 to 1. Being a woman you need to be even more careful about your scoliosis because the condition is expected to progressively increase at a faster rate. The ratio of females to males who have a curve greater than 30 degrees is even more skewed to the order of 10 to 1. As a woman, you are also eight times more likely to develop a curve that requires immediate and focused attention.

If you have been diagnosed with scoliosis, then chances are that you may already be taking some kind of treatment. Make sure that you are following what is best for you and your baby at the time of pregnancy in order to avoid any kind of medication, physical therapy or surgery that will make things worse.

It is also true that many scoliosis cases (approximately four out of five) have a curve in the spine that is less than 20 degrees. Such curve levels are not noticed on casual examination and may therefore be overlooked in most cases. They are also not prominent enough when you stand, walk or sit. If you have reached skeletal maturity then you do not have to get such minor curvatures treated.

However, when you are pregnant, even smaller curves up to 20-degrees may also lead to a higher level of problems. If you have a doubt about your condition and suspect that you may have scoliosis, then you must get it checked and diagnosed so that you can take the required precautions to make your journey to childbirth easier. There are exercises that you can do to make the entire nine months more bearable. There is also a scoliosis friendly diet (discussed in Chapter 11) that ensures that you get all the nutrients that can help you keep your spine and baby happy and healthy.

If your scoliosis was diagnosed when you were in your teens, it will pay to have your scoliosis checked regularly. This is because it is unlikely that you would have reached skeletal maturity at that age and therefore the chances of the curve having increased since then are high.

Sometimes scoliosis is confused with kyphosis, which is an abnormal curve of the spine that can be seen from the side. This means that when you see the spine from the front, it will appear to be normal as the curve is not visible from this angle. The spine can bend forward in an abnormal manner giving the person a hunched posture. The emphasis is on the word abnormal because the spine bends and curves naturally from front to back in the middle part of the spine called the thoracic spine.

Another condition that is also confused with scoliosis is lordosis. This is mainly because the conditions are similar and are related to the curvatures of the spine. Like in kyphosis, the curve in lordosis can only be seen from the side. If you look at the spine x-ray from the front or the rear, the spine will appear to be in a straight line. The abnormal curve can only be seen from the side and the spine seems to be bent backwards in an abnormal way. Here again the normal curve backwards of the spine that is seen in the upper spinal area called the cervical or the lower spine area called the lumbar is not to be mistaken as lordosis.

If you have scoliosis and are worried about how to manage it, you need not fret. The fact that you are reading this book points towards the positive attitude that you have towards your scoliosis and that you are curious to find out more about the various treatment and therapy options that exist.

Typically scoliosis is treated using various options like exercise therapy, bracing and surgery. Some holistic physicians also ensure that their patients consume a good healthy diet that can help the spine develop normally and remain healthy. This has been explained in my first book, "Your Plan for Natural Scoliosis Prevention and Treatment". The holistic approach is often a good option for those who are pregnant because the treatment is great for children as well. The holistic approach may also help reduce the chances of your baby developing congenital scoliosis.

When you go to your doctor with concerns about your scoliosis condition, you should know the specific signs and symptoms that you have. This means that you need to be aware of the specifications of your scoliosis to the extent that you can be. It is also important for expectant mothers with scoliosis to know these symptoms because she may be able to identify it in her child at an earlier stage in case the condition has passed on genetically.

Scoliosis is a condition that is associated with the genes and therefore it is necessary that mothers with scoliosis be more aware of the factors that cause it. Since there is a higher chance of your child developing the condition you have, knowing the factors that can potentially trigger the scoliosis can help you prevent it in many cases.

The school screening process can also help you because it can detect scoliosis at an early stage. The average adolescent scoliosis is about 30 degrees and it is expected to increase by 7 degrees with each passing year if it is not controlled. When you are able to detect the scoliosis early you shall be able to keep the progression under control; something that is especially important for girls because the progression is expected to be higher in them.

In addition, there are different kinds of scoliosis that people may have. If you are able to identify the kind of scoliosis you have you will be able to manage the condition better. This can help you take better care of yourself when you are pregnant too. Some of the types of scoliosis are listed below. Sometimes people do not fit into just one kind of scoliosis and may span different types.

- *Congenital scoliosis* — This kind of scoliosis is a vertebral abnormality that someone is born with.

- *Idiopathic scoliosis* — This kind of scoliosis occurs without any known reason. Most cases of scoliosis are categorized as idiopathic scoliosis because the real reason for the condition is not yet known. Many infantile, juvenile, adolescent or adult scoliosis are classified as idiopathic if there is no specific factor, disease, condition or event that may have caused it. It is estimated that about 80 percent of the scoliosis cases are idiopathic and most of these occur in adolescent females. When the condition occurs before the age of 3 years, it is called infantile idiopathic scoliosis. If the scoliosis is diagnosed between ages 3 and 10, it is referred to as juvenile idiopathic scoliosis and those after the age of 10 are called adolescent idiopathic scoliosis.

- *Neuromuscular scoliosis* — In some cases people tend to develop a curve in their spine due to another medical disease. In most cases, it is a secondary symptom of another medical condition. If someone has a condition that leads to poor muscle control or weakness in the muscles, the chances of scoliosis are large. Spina bifida, spinal muscular atrophy, cerebral palsy, Marfan's disease or physical trauma or shock are some conditions that have been associated with scoliosis in many cases. Neuromuscular scoliosis is usually extremely severe and invariably requires aggressive treatment.

- *Degenerative scoliosis* — When scoliosis is first detected among adults, it is generally degenerative scoliosis. This kind of scoliosis occurs due to a variety of other factors such as arthritis, spondylitis or weakening of the ligaments, soft tissues and muscles that support the back. Some other factors that may cause this type of scoliosis include osteoporosis, disc degeneration and vertebral compression fractures. In some cases it may also be caused due to excessive bad posture and poor lifestyle.

- *Functional scoliosis* — Functional scoliosis can be caused due to some other kind of deformity in another part of the body. A shorter leg or muscle spasms in the back can lead to scoliosis of this kind.

- *Other causes of scoliosis* — Sometimes scoliosis is also known to be caused due to spine tumors such as osteoid osteoma; a benign tumor that generally occurs in the spine and causes immense back pain. The pain is the main reason why people tend to adopt a more comfortable stance, thereby leading to bending of back towards one side. Over time, this causes a deformity in the spine leading to scoliosis.

CHAPTER 2

FACTORS THAT CAUSE SCOLIOSIS

Among the many diseases that researchers and medical professionals do not yet understand completely is scoliosis. The exact reasons for idiopathic scoliosis have not been found till date. However, there is nothing to be apprehensive about because there are some factors that are known to play a significant role in scoliosis. Some of the factors that doctors feel may influence the presence, onset or progression of scoliosis include hormonal imbalances, mechanical or genetic defects and poor nutrition.

There are research studies being conducted even as you read this book to understand the specific reasons for the abnormality of the curve of your spine. Some scholars feel that understanding the various accompanying conditions can give us a better understanding of the factors that can cause scoliosis. Scholars have studied these conditions and discovered some of the major likely reasons that can cause scoliosis. So, even when we do not know the exact factors that lead to scoliosis, knowing about the various factors that are being considered as causes of scoliosis can help us ensure that the scoliosis does not occur or that the progression can be controlled. You may be able to ensure a healthier baby who has a lower chance of getting scoliosis, even if you suffer from the condition yourself, by ensuring that you prevent some of these risk factors in your life.

Magnesium deficiency is the first thing that needs to be mentioned when we look at the probable causes of scoliosis. Many people who have the heart condition called Mitral Valve Prolapse (MVP) are also prone to scoliosis. A study conducted in India showed that 55 percent of children diagnosed with Mitral Valve Prolapse also had scoliosis. MVP is also considered similar to scoliosis because it is also more common among women than in men. The symptoms of both these conditions aggravate at the time of puberty.

Dr. Roger J. Williams, one of the earliest proponents of Metabolic Typing and author of the revolutionary book 'Biochemical Individuality' has mentioned that diets that are adequate for young children are not sufficient for adolescents, especially those entering puberty. If the diet does not change in line with the changing requirements of the body at that time, various deficiencies can occur. It has also been seen that as high as 85 percent of those who have been diagnosed with Mitral Valve Prolapse are magnesium deficient too. There have also been studies where patients with MVP were provided with magnesium supplement and the results showed symptomatic relief of the patients.

In addition, magnesium deficiency has also been identified as a cause of osteoporosis and osteopenia, two other conditions that are largely linked with scoliosis. It is also known that lack of adequate levels of magnesium in the body can cause muscle contractions, an issue that we already know can lead to scoliosis.

Vitamin K is the other nutrient that has a significant effect on the presence of scoliosis. Many studies have already been done that tell us that a vitamin K deficiency is associated with excessive bleeding as seen in heavy or prolonged menstrual bleeding. Some of the other issues that vitamin K deficiency can cause include blood in the urine (hematuria), bruising, gastrointestinal bleeding, nose-bleeds and more. This condition is also associated with osteoporosis, another condition that often occurs along with scoliosis.

Hypo-estrogenism or low estrogen levels have also been linked to scoliosis. If you have low levels of estrogen, you are more likely to have osteoporosis and osteopenia, two conditions that often accompany scoliosis.

Women who maintain a low body weight due to their professional requirement or otherwise, tend to have low estrogen levels. Various studies done among these women who maintain a low body weight in order to remain slim have shown a higher incidence of scoliosis in them. For example, a study among ballet dancers showed that they were more prone to scoliosis and stress fractures up to an incidence of between 24 and 40 percent. In one of the studies, the incidence rate of scoliosis among rhythmic gymnasts as compared to a control group was 10 times higher. Female athletes are also known to have a higher rate of scoliosis than women in general. Some of the other aspects associated with hypo-estrogenism include fractures, double joints, delayed puberty and low body weight.

Vitamin D and zinc deficiency have also been associated with the probability of getting scoliosis. People who maintain a diet that is low in zinc and vitamin D tend to have a sunken chest condition. This is medically called pectus excavatum; another condition that occurs commonly with scoliosis.

To summarize, deficiencies in magnesium, zinc, vitamin K, vitamin D, selenium and low levels of estrogen can lead to a higher probability of getting scoliosis. Some scholars also believe that scoliosis is linked to genetic inheritance. This is also a generally accepted causative factor. While research on this continues, the CHD7 gene has been associated with the presence of scoliosis at birth.

The hypothesis that scoliosis is a genetic condition could be ascertained by the fact that if you have a relative who has scoliosis, there is a 25 percent to 35 percent chance that you will also have the same condition6. If both your parents have the condition there is a 40 percent chance that you will have it. If you and your partner have scoliosis, then there is a similar 40 percent chance that your child will have it as well. However, taking some precautions, like ensuring a nutritious diet that is good for scoliosis before pregnancy, during pregnancy as well as post-delivery can help reduce the chances of your baby confer the same condition.

However, it is also known that identical twins may not always share the condition all the time. This shows that scoliosis can be caused by other non-genetic factors as well.

As parents you have a duty to perform by understanding all that there is to know about the condition in order to make sure that you do everything in your power to reduce the chances of passing it on to your children. You need to be extra vigilant about the symptoms of scoliosis among your children so that you can catch the situation early in life and keep it from progressing further. Make sure that you have regular check-ups for your children. Make exercise a daily family routine so that you can keep the spine healthy and fit. Follow a scoliosis friendly diet (as detailed later in chapter 11) so that the entire family can stay healthy and lead a comfortable life.

Having treated a large number of scoliosis patients for many years, I have come across many people who ask whether their scoliosis has been caused by sleeping in the wrong position, lifting heavy weights or putting undue strain on their muscles. While these may seem like logical causes of scoliosis, it is not indeed so. However, if you suffer from scoliosis and a curved spine you may experience higher levels of pain, discomfort and strain when lifting heavy weights or sleeping in certain positions.

While researchers may still be trying to find out a single cause for scoliosis, the fact remains that it is a medical condition that can be caused due to various factors. It is now widely accepted that scoliosis patients have some abnormality in structural, neurological, biochemical or genetic makeup that really causes scoliosis.

Over time and after having looked at the entire medical histories of thousands of scoliosis patients, I have come to believe that one or more among the following factors, such as defective genes, unnatural biochemical forces, poor diet and inadequate nutrition, physical asymmetry, issues in the brain and hormonal imbalances that cause estrogen deficiency may lead to scoliosis.

CHAPTER 3

SCOLIOSIS AND PREGNANCY THE CONNECTION

First things first, scoliosis is not a condition that should prevent you from enjoying the joys of motherhood. If you have scoliosis, there is no need to worry about anything or deprive yourself from getting pregnant. All that you have to understand is that scoliosis is linked to genes and therefore there is a relatively higher chance of your child getting the condition than someone else whose parents do not have scoliosis.

Another aspect that you need to keep in mind is that if you have a curved spine, there is an extra care that you may need to take during pregnancy and post-delivery period to ensure that you do not harm yourself in the process. This is necessary because the baby does put some pressure on the spine and you will have to be extra cautious to ensure that you and your baby both remain safe during the course of the pregnancy.

Most researchers believe that scoliosis has a significant connection with genes. This is mainly the case because a large number of idiopathic and congenital cases are seen every year. Just as your genes are responsible for the way you look, the way you behave, specific things that you feel, they also define the specific diseases to which we are predisposed. These genes elevate the risk for specific kinds of diseases.

Yes, there is a genetic link for scoliosis. However, this does not mean that every child born to a mother who has scoliosis will have the same condition. It is heartening to know that while our children have the genes that we pass on to them it does not mean that we have no control over them whatsoever. While you cannot change your genes, you can manage the way in which these genes express themselves. Genes can be literally turned off or on by various environmental factors, nutrition, foods and lifestyle too. In this way, we can reduce the negative effects that some genes have on our body and mind. Genetic testing became available to the public in 2009. There is however a lot of research that still needs to be done in this area. At the same time much has already been achieved too. Concerning scoliosis, we understand the manner in which specific genes affect curve progression. This is a great discovery for us to be able to assess whether surgery is required or not. It also helps us understand the level to which we can manage the condition with diet, proper nutrition and exercise.

Does genetics offer help?

Interestingly, genetics premises new hope for patients of scoliosis, though the research for expectant mothers with scoliosis is still underway.

However, in a few types, such as the congenital forms of scoliosis, prenatal genetic testing can point out towards conditions such as neurofibromatosis, muscular dystrophy and some types of myopathy. In addition, the routine ultrasound scans done at various stages of pregnancy can also check for any abnormalities in the pattern of the spinal growth of the fetus.

Nevertheless, experts point out that since multiple occurrences in a single family are not very common, the likelihood that a mother with scoliosis will pass it on is quite less likely.

A genome wide study was conducted in this area and it was found that there are nucleotide polymorphism markers that are present in the DNA. These have been associated with adolescent idiopathic scoliosis. Fifty three such genetic markers have been identified and scoliosis has been termed as a biomechanical deformity. It has also been suggested that the rate and level of progression depends on the asymmetric forces according to Hueter-Volkmann law, which states that remodeling of the spine may occur because of gravitational stresses and asymmetrical forces.

While the health of the baby is one issue that is of concern when a mother has scoliosis, another is that many pregnant women worry about their health post-delivery. You may be worried about how the scoliosis will be affected due to the pregnancy and the manner in which the delivery will harm the spinal curve that you have. It is a good thing that you are thinking about these things because there are some precautions that you shall take in order to ensure a safe and easy delivery. However, there is no reason to be apprehensive about it because it is possible, even with scoliosis, to have a normal and health delivery and give birth to a healthy child. While your child will be at a higher risk of developing scoliosis, there are various nutritional therapies that can help reduce the chances of scoliosis. If you are aware about your scoliosis and take all the precautions about the kind of foods that you eat during your pregnancy, you might be able to prevent this condition in your baby completely.

Our body has trillions of cells and each cell has a DNA that is basically the genetic code that we all carry. We know that it takes many generations to change this code or 'rewrite' this basic code. On top of the genes there are chemicals called epigenetic markers. These chemicals are responsible for providing instructions to the genes. In this manner they are able to activate specific genes and silence others. What is really interesting to note is that specific foods that you eat can lead to the activation of the epigenetic markers that can in turn activate or deactivate specific genes. What this means for scoliotic mothers is that if you eat the right food, you can ensure that the epigenetic markers that lead to activation of the gene that controls scoliosis are not triggered off; thereby ensuring that the genes are not passed on to the unborn offspring.

The study conducted at Medical Genetics Institute at Cedars-Sinai Medical Center showed that scoliosis could be caused due to mutations of a specific gene as well. The same study also showed that adequate levels of calcium are necessary for proper spine development when the fetus is developing in the womb. This study gave us ample reason to believe that nutrition plays an essential role in the probability of getting scoliosis even among those who are otherwise genetically predisposed to it.

All researches and evidence shows that even women who have scoliosis can have a regular pregnancy.

A relevant survey carried out by Phillip Zorab and Dr David Siegler amongst 64 women with scoliosis found that these women encountered no serious medical complications. Though 17% of mothers reported increased breathlessness and 21% had increased back pain, yet both the groups found it manageable enough. Meanwhile, a normal delivery was carried out for most women with only 17% requiring a caesarean section, that too for obstetric reasons .

Nevertheless, the fact remains that pregnant women are more prone to higher levels of progression of scoliosis than those who are not. It is therefore necessary that you take extra care concerning your nutrition, diet, exercises, postures, sleeping positions and delivery positions. Learning about these aspects can make all the difference in terms of having a normal, healthy and easy pregnancy.

In addition to that, it has been noted that women who are careful about the above mentioned aspects do not face as many complications post-delivery as do those who are not.

Some women tend to feel that they need to undergo surgery in order to correct their scoliosis and then conceive. This is not necessary if you are aware about the ScoliScore AIS Prognostic Test. This new genetic test looks at the DNA of Adolescent Idiopathic Scoliosis patients and detects the probability of spinal curve progression. This test can help physicians understand whether surgery will ever be required for the patient or not. A large number of people (about 85 to 90 percent) who are diagnosed with Adolescent Idiopathic Scoliosis (AIS) do not need surgery for their mild curve. This means that if your scoliosis has a Cobb's angle between 10 and 25 degree, you need not worry about interventions and surgery. Proper exercise and a good diet can ensure a healthy life for you and your baby. These tests have been proved to be accurate 99 percent of the time and therefore are extremely reliable.

All this said, you need to know that there is a possibility that pregnancy may exaggerate your scoliosis curve to some extent. The manner in which your pregnancy takes course will decide whether you can have a normal delivery or whether you will need to undergo a Caesarean section. In some cases, there are complications that may arise in administering an epidural anesthesia. However, these are not complications that a good anesthesiologist and a proficient gynecologist cannot handle.

What is a Cobb Angle?

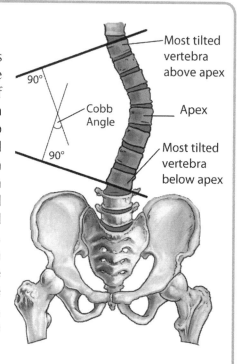

The term "Cobb Angle" is used worldwide to measure and quantify the magnitude of spinal deformities, especially in the case of scoliosis. The Cobb angle measurement is the "gold standard" of scoliosis evaluation endorsed by Scoliosis Research Society. It is used as the standard measurement to quantify and track the progression of scoliosis. Cobb angle was first described in 1948 by Dr. John R Cobb where he outlined how to measure the angle of the spinal curve. Hence, the term "Cobb Angle" came about, bearing his name.

How to measure a Cobb Angle?

An X-ray is needed to measure the Cobb angle.

1. Locate the most tilted vertebra at the top of the curve and draw a parallel line to the superior vertebral end plate.

2. Locate the most tilted vertebra at the bottom of the curve and draw a parallel line to the inferior vertebral end plate.

3. Erect intersecting perpendicular lines from the two parallel lines.

4. The angle formed between the two parallel lines is Cobb angle.

CHAPTER 4

SYMPTOMS, DIAGNOSIS AND COMPLICATIONS IN SCOLIOSIS

Understanding the signs and symptoms of scoliosis is essential for two reasons. Firstly, it helps you assess the level of scoliosis that you have so that you can adjust your lifestyle accordingly. On the other hand, as a mother who has scoliosis, you will need to know these signs and symptoms in order to assess whether your child is developing it or not.

A curved spinal cord can lead to a large number of other complications and if the condition is identified at a stage where the curve progression has not increased to a high level, there are various procedures and therapies that can prevent the curve from progressing faster than otherwise. Once identified, the condition can be treated using diet, exercise and other natural treatment options so that you can maintain a healthy lifestyle and live a fuller life.

Symptoms of Scoliosis

Below are some of the common symptoms of scoliosis. These symptoms will help you identify the condition when you see it. It will help you understand the exercises detailed later in this book and do it in the right manner. Take a look at these and then try to assess whether you have any of these symptoms to determine whether you have scoliosis or not.

- Trunk or neck deviated to one side

- Uneven musculature on one side

- Prominent shoulder blade on one side

- Rib prominence

- Uneven hips

- Uneven length of the legs

- Backache or pain in the low back

- Fatigue

- Difficulty in sitting or standing in one position for a long time

- Difficulty in breathing (if the curve in the spine is extremely large and more than 70 degrees)

While you can assess the symptoms of scoliosis at home it is a good idea to get this checked by a physician. While it is possible for a physician to miss a slight curve during a routine physical examination, when you go for a scoliosis-check specifically, you will obviously undergo the confirmatory tests that are required to determine whether you have scoliosis or not.

Scoliosis often starts with a sight curve in the spine that may be missed during regular visits to the doctor where the physician may not specifically look for a curved spine. When you have a curve level of 10 to 20 degrees, chances are that there will be no overt manifestations of the same. You may not really be able to perceive an uneven shoulder or an uneven hip joint level on your own.

The scoliosis curve is expected to increase until skeletal maturity is reached. The rate at which the progression takes place depends on various factors including genes, environment, nutrition and lifestyle.

In many cases scoliosis is discovered when friends or relatives notice a slight deviation at the level of the hips or the shoulders. Since the changes in the spinal curve are insidious, it is often easy to miss such progression. If you have a progressing scoliosis you may notice that clothes that used to fit you perfectly do not seem to fit as well. In some cases you may notice that the legs of pants are longer on one side.

Curves below 10 degrees are considered mild and therefore medical professionals do not prescribe any specific mode of treatment. This level of curve can straighten itself if adequate care is taken with posture, exercise and diet. Less than a third of such mild scoliosis develops into higher degrees of curve that require treatment. Curves that are diagnosed at around 30 degrees are more likely to progress.

However, if you have mild scoliosis and are aware of the things that you need to do in order to control the progression, you will be in a better situation a few years down the line. If you heed proper nutrition guidelines that promote better spine health you will be able to manage the progression of the curve in a better manner. By doing this you will also ensure that you are limiting the chances of this becoming a bigger concern at a later date.

Scoliosis Complications

A large number of medical conditions have been associated closely with scoliosis. In addition to the various complications that can arise, the presence of scoliosis also indicates that you are at a higher risk for the other associated medical conditions as well. This means that you need to guard against them in order to remain healthy.

Some of the health conditions that have been associated with scoliosis include the following:

- *Ehler-Danlos syndrome* — Sometimes called the floppy baby syndrome, this is a connective tissue disorder that is generally caused by an inability to synthesize collagen properly.

- *Charcot-Marie-Tooth* — An inherited condition that is characterized by loss of the muscle tissue and loss of sensation.

- *Prader-Willi Syndrome* — A disease that is considered rare, this is a condition in which seven genes are undetected, unexpressed or missing. It causes a delay in speech, lack of physical coordination, weight gain and sleep disorders. It can lead to delayed puberty or infertility as well.

- *Cerebral Palsy* — A condition associated with the cerebrum that includes a range of specific motor disability issues. This condition is classified as spastic, ataxic, dyskinetic and hypotonic.

- *Spinal Muscular Atrophy* — A disease, linked to the nerves and the muscles that leads to muscular weakness and atrophy.

- *Muscular Dystrophy* — This is a muscle disease and is also considered hereditary. It manifests itself in the form of muscle weakness, defects in muscle protein and death of muscle cells and tissue.

- *CHARGE Syndrome* — This is a genetic disorder that is associated with Coloboma of the eye, defects in the heart, atresia of the nasal choanae, retardation, genital abnormalities, yeast infections and deafness.

- *Familial Dysautonomia* — Also called Riley-Day Syndrome, this is a condition related to the autonomous nervous system. It results in insensitivity to pain, poor growth, inability to produce tears and more.

- *Friedreich's Ataxia* — Another inherited condition that leads to speech issues, gait disorders, heart diseases and diabetes.

- *Proteus Syndrome* — Also called Wiedemann's syndrome, this condition can cause abnormal bone development, skin overgrowth and tumors in the body.

- *Spina Bifida* — A congenital disorder that results from the incomplete closing of the embryonic neural tube.

- *Marfan's Syndrome* — A connective tissue disorder, this is also a genetic disorder that can affect the skeletal system, the heart, the eyes and the central nervous system.

- *Neurofibromatosis* — A condition where nervous tissue tumors can cause an array of nerve related disorders.

- *Congenital Diaphragmatic Hernia* — This condition refers to a birth defect of the diaphragm.

- *Hemi-hypertrophy* — A condition where one side of the body is larger than the other, this condition can lead to a higher risk of specific types of cancer.

While this looks like a long and scary list, these are rare and not always present if you have scoliosis. The list has been placed here to give you an idea of the various conditions that you may need to watch out for since they are closely related with scoliosis.

Even if you have scoliosis, chances are that you will live your life without the need of surgical intervention. This means that you will not have to go under the scalpel and expose yourself to all the risks that it carries. However, about 5 percent of those who do have scoliosis tend to need surgery to be able to perform their daily duties adequately. Surgery does have a risk of inflammation of the soft tissues. It has also been known to cause breathing disablement, nerve injuries and internal bleeding in some cases. If you are considering surgery, think about some of the latest statistics: About 5 percent of those who undergo scoliosis surgery get a relapse of sorts within 5 years of the procedure. This indicates that the predisposition to scoliosis is not something that vanishes as soon as you get it corrected surgically. In addition, many researchers feel that correcting the spine surgically is not possible and that the procedure is merely superficial and cosmetic.

Besides these physical complications that scoliosis can cause, there are also various concerns that people face in terms of trauma. In the severe form, the condition can lead to a life of limited activity. Young people may find it extremely uncomfortable and embarrassing to wear a brace in public. The pain, limited activity and the obvious display of their deformity can lead many people to depression. As an aware person you need to battle the condition with courage. There is no need to worry about these aspects and you can rest assured that with the right kind of nutrition, diet and the exercises, the condition can be controlled and managed.

Diagnosis

If someone in your family has scoliosis, it is pertinent that you look out for the condition in the children of the household. A simple test can be done at home to determine whether your child has scoliosis or not and whether you need to visit a physician to get a confirmation.

This is what you need to do in order to help you decide whether you need to go to a doctor to confirm the presence of scoliosis. You will need a pen and paper so that you can record the observations you make. You will also need paper dots that have adhesive to marks positions on the body. Then follow the steps detailed below.

1. Ask your child to bend forward and place an adhesive dot on the bones of the spine that can be felt along the back. These can also be seen easily when a person is bending forward. To make sure that you have done this correctly, check that you have six dots on the back of the neck, 12 dots on the mid back and five dots on the lower back. You should therefore have 23 dots in all. You may find that you have not been able to place all 23 dots. Do not worry or panic about this because it is not always possible to find all the spine bones that stick out. This also does not mean anything as far as scoliosis diagnosis is concerned and therefore you need not assume anything at this stage.

2. Ask your child to stand straight and be relaxed. Look at the row of dots to see if they appear in a straight line. If the line of dots seems crooked or curved at any place, make a note. It helps to draw a single diagram of a human body structure and make note of the specific areas where the curves appear.

3. Also look for specific aspects such as

    a. Is one shoulder high or low — If yes, which one?

    b. Do the ribs appear higher on one side — If yes, which side is higher?

    c. Does one shoulder blade protrude out more than the other — If yes, which shoulder?

    d. Is one hip higher than the other — If yes, which one?

    e.   Does the lower back protrude outwards on one side —
If yes, which side?

4. Ask your child to bend forwards while keeping the palms together. Look for the specific aspects mentioned above and note them on a piece of paper again.

If you have not observed a shoulder higher than another, an uneven protuberance of the shoulder blades, one hip higher than the other, prominent rib cage on one side, an uneven lower back or a crooked line of dots, then there is nothing to worry about. On the other hand, if you have noticed that most of these things appear in the case of your child you need to confirm these with a trained physician. In case you have noticed a couple of things from the many observations listed above, you may still want to visit a professional medical doctor in order to remove any doubts about your observation. It may be possible that your child has mild scoliosis that you have not been able to perceive correctly. Taking such a precaution is better than leaving it alone and allowing the curve to progress further without any kind of treatment.

Even a doctor with a keen eye may miss a mild scoliotic curve unless he is looking for it specifically. This is why it is important that you ask specifically for a scoliosis examination if there is someone in your family who suffers from this condition.

When you go for a check-up for scoliosis, the physician is likely to ask you many questions concerning your family history. Other questions pertaining to weakness, muscle pain, restriction of activities are also to be expected.

Next, you may be asked to undress from the waist up and bend forward. This helps in identifying the nature of the curve of the spine. This is called the Adams Forward Bend Test. The test requires you to dangle your arms while keeping your knees straight. This allows the doctor to appreciate and examine the curve, the symmetry of the body, the shoulders, the hips and the rib cage more easily. Range of motion, muscle strength and reflexes are also generally checked at this stage of visit. If this is your first visit to the doctor, he may note your height and weight in order to be able to assess the extent of progress if he notices a slight curve. This test however, is not fool-proof. It has been known to miss a large number of lower back scoliosis and 15 percent of the scoliosis cases in general. So, while this is a reliable screening test, it should not be used as the final judgment without checking any further.

In some cases Scoliometer screening is done. This is carried out by using a device that measures the extent of the curve of the spine. You can also use ScolioTrack for iPad, iPhone or Android devices. It is an innovative way to track the scoliosis condition in the comfort of your home just as a doctor would in his office. With this application, you do not need to go through expensive and time consuming x-rays at the doctor's clinic. You can even document the manner in which the scoliosis progression takes place. You can download this application using any smart phone. For more information about the ScolioTrack, check the resources section of the book.

At this stage if the physician suspects scoliosis, a whole spine weight bearing x-ray is asked for. This is done in two planes, the frontal or back view and the lateral or sagittal view. Depending on the severity of the curve on initial x-rays, you may need to get this repeated every three months or every year as recommended by the physician. This is mainly done to check the progression of the curve.

The Cobb's Angle measurement is used to quantify the severity of the curve in the spine. The angle is measured from the upper end-plate of the top-most vertebrae to the lower end-plate of the lower-most vertebrae involved. In some cases this needs to be done at two locations in the spine if the curves are multiple.

Adams Forward Bend Test

The forward bend test is a test used most often in schools and doctor's offices to screen for scoliosis. During the test, the child bends forward with the feet together and knees straight while dangling the arms. Any imbalances in the rib cage or other deformities along the back could be a sign of scoliosis.

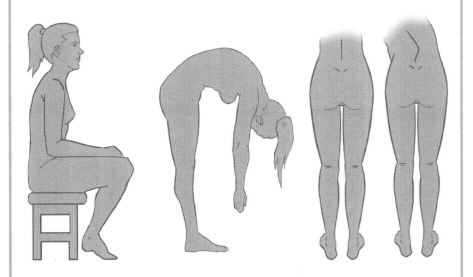

The forward bend test, however, is not sensitive to abnormalities in the lower back, a very common site for scoliosis. Because the test misses about 15% of scoliosis cases, many experts do not recommend it as the sole method for screening for scoliosis.

CHAPTER 5

HEALTH CONSEQUENCES OF SCOLIOSIS

Now that we know what scoliosis is all about, the various factors that can cause the condition, its symptoms and likelihood of passing the condition on to your child, we should look at the health consequences of scoliosis in detail.

The association of scoliosis and pregnancy and the concerns about being pregnant with scoliosis are obvious. We all know that carrying a child is not an easy task. The mother has to live with a life inside her for a period of nine months with the latter part of the term becoming extremely difficult to manage in terms of the additional weight that one needs to carry around in the body.

Most expecting mothers worry about the manner in which their condition will worsen due to the pregnancy, the trauma that they might have to go through during delivery and the effect that their condition will have on their baby. Before 1950, it was believed extensively that pregnancy could cause the curve of the scoliosis to increase significantly. In fact, it was also believed that scoliosis reduces fertility to a large extent. Studies have shown over time that neither of this is true.

Some feel that the curve of the spine will increase further with the additional weight that needs to be carried for such a long period of time. You may also feel that the expanded uterus will put pressure on various parts of the body and result in a situation where the scoliosis condition will worsen over time. Most of us know that the alterations in the body cause women to have various issues and backache is one of the most common concerns in the third trimester. The fear about pregnancy leaving you with a chronic backache condition is common.

While there are some complications that pregnancy can cause in women having scoliosis, a lot depends on the severity of the scoliosis and the manner in which you handle your pregnancy. Mild cases of scoliosis can go through the entire pregnancy without really having any issues that are any different from an ordinary pregnancy. All that you may need to worry about if you have mild scoliosis is the diet that you consume and certain specific exercises. These are the concerns that all pregnant women should take into consideration.

However, in some cases where the scoliosis is moderate or severe, you may experience back pain to a higher level than normal. As it is, research shows that almost 80% of the people are likely to have a back pain sometime in their life. Hence, it is natural in the case of pregnant women, since the growth of the baby affects the mother's posture while the abdominal muscles stretch up to their maximum limit to make way for the baby. This is something that is likely to continue from the latter half of the second trimester till delivery, maybe even later. However, the good news is that there are ways you can ensure that backaches are managed well and kept under control with the right exercises.

Those who suffer from severe scoliosis may have issues with breathlessness and other kinds of breathing trouble. This is something that you may experience towards the third trimester when the baby is large and starts to push against the diaphragm. Here again, this is a condition that many women face as they enter the third trimester. Though, it may be more prominent and conspicuous in your case. This means that it needs more concentrated and focused handling in order to ensure that you do not experience any breathing issues. Refer to the section on details of the last trimester for further details on this.

Pain management, therefore, becomes an important and critical aspect of pregnancy with scoliosis. It is something that you will have to consider much before the actual delivery because the pain can get tough to handle when bearing the baby as well.

The delivery process may be different if you have severe scoliosis. Some are lucky enough to go through a normal delivery despite the scoliosis, depending on the curve and the severity of the condition. However, others may have to get an epidural and even a caesarean section. The final decision concerning the specific kind of delivery that you should have depends on your doctor and shall be made based on your health, the babies' comfort during delivery, the level and curve of scoliosis and other complications involved. Many women have discovered that it is very much possible to have a normal vaginal delivery despite having scoliosis.

The one thing that you do need to remember is that you should be informed and aware of your scoliosis condition and that you should mention this to your gynecologist during your first visit. This will ensure that your gynecologist consults a trained professional or a chiropractor concerning the manner in which the pregnancy should be taken forward and the specific precautions that need to be taken in order to ensure a safe and healthy pregnancy for you and your baby.

For those who have had a surgery to correct scoliosis, you will need to wait for around six months to a year before trying to conceive. This is because the body needs to heal before it can take the burden that comes along with being pregnant. You should also consult your doctor before you start the process of conception because each case is different and needs to be treated individually.

Having said all this, it is important to remember that a history of scoliosis does not increase the risk of curve progression unless you have extremely severe scoliosis and if you have not been taking the right precautions concerning your lifestyle, nutrition and exercise. For someone who is prone to osteoporosis or degenerative disc disease, sitting in one place for too long can predispose you to develop scoliosis.

A study conducted among 355 women affected with scoliosis who had reached skeletal maturity (Risser Grade 4) were studied and analyzed. These women were divided into two groups. Group A consisted of 175 women who had had at least one pregnancy. Group B consisted of 180 women who had never been pregnant. These groups were matched in terms of the kind of treatment that they had received for their scoliosis. It was noted that the curve progressed in both the groups to some extent. The extent of the progression was more than 5 degrees in 25 percent of the women and greater than 10 degrees in about 10 percent. However, this is something that was noted in both the groups to a similar extent. This study showed that the level of curve progression could not be attributed to the pregnancy at all.

It was also noted that the age of the women at the time of pregnancy did not affect the progression. When the delivery histories of the women in Group A were studied there were no signs of any complication throughout the delivery process, except for four women who faced difficulty in delivery. There were some cases of caesarean section delivery, but these were not related to scoliosis in any manner.

Back pain is one aspect of pregnancy that needs to be managed thoroughly. This is something that has been seen in about 50 percent of the cases of pregnant women with scoliosis. The management of the pain depends on whether the pain is lumbar or sacroiliac in nature. Specific exercises, reduced mobility, use of a wheel chair in the latter months and other therapies are recognized modalities for managing the condition and are thereby encouraged.

While there are no specific drugs to treat scoliosis, there are some of you who may be taking some pain relief medication. If you are taking some drugs in order to treat scoliosis, it is pertinent that you consult your gynecologist about these. Some of these drugs are now known to cause birth defects in children and you need to be aware of these even before you think about conception. It is always best to stop such medication a few months before you think of having a baby rather than to repent later.

Another aspect that you need to be careful about when you are planning a pregnancy with scoliosis is your bowel and bladder issues. Those who have some concerns about the bowel and bladder movements may realize that the condition exaggerates during pregnancy. Sometimes it also results in an inability to push during the delivery process causing a forced suction or forceps delivery.

The one thing that you do not have to worry about is what the baby goes through during delivery if you have scoliosis. In a large number of cases, the specific type of delivery is based on factors other than scoliosis. These could be either breech position of your baby or a non-expanding cervix. Seldom do you find a situation where a caesarean section has been performed solely because the mother has scoliosis.

The chances of your child having congenital scoliosis are not higher if you have the condition yourself. However, there is a higher likelihood your child may get an idiopathic scoliosis and this is something that you will need to be aware of as the years advance.

CHAPTER 6

CONVENTIONAL SCOLIOSIS TREATMENTS

The treatment options that your physician may suggest depend on various factors that include aspects such as the extent of curvature, gender, age, whether you have reached skeletal maturity, general health conditions and the location of the curve.

Depending on the severity of scoliosis you have in terms of the curve, you may be able to continue your life without any issues at all. However, it is known that scoliosis can cause a reduction in life expectancy by an average of 14 years. In addition, we also know that scoliosis can cause additional complications during pregnancy, even though it does not stop you from having a normal delivery. There are complications that one needs to be aware of and prevent in order to be able to have a safe pregnancy.

Many doctors tend to suggest the "wait and watch" approach for scoliosis. This is because there is no conventional permanent cure for scoliosis that you are likely to get from your modern day medicine professional. For mild scoliosis, the doctor is likely to recommend that you regularly monitor the curve and continue to get check-ups and x-rays to watch the progression.

In all probability, if you have a curve that is larger than 25 degrees you may be advised to wear a brace and in more severe cases above 40 degrees, you may even land up in the operation room. While these options are discussed in detail below, you do have to remember that you can still prevent the progression of scoliosis if you already suffer from the condition. You can also benefit from a treatment or therapy option that allows you to reduce the chances of passing on the same to your offspring.

The lack of options for treatment from doctors is not surprising. The fact is that they are not aware of any regular treatment option that can help in curing the scoliosis completely. This stems from the fact that a large proportion of diagnosed scoliosis is idiopathic in nature. Till date doctors are not aware of what causes the abnormal spine curvature to occur. They can only guess whether the scoliosis curve is due to an underdeveloped skeletal framework, an incapable connective tissue or other genetic or environmental influences that trigger a curve to appear.

In the cases where the physician recommends an active treatment option, bracing is the most commonly prescribed. There are various kinds of braces that are present and these are mostly named after the centers where they were developed. The choice of brace to use in your case shall be decided based on the extent and location of the curve you have. Some of the commonly used types of braces are:

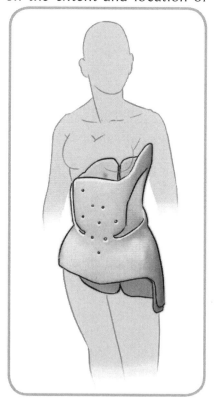

- *The Boston Brace* — Also called the Thoraco-Lumbo-Sacral-Orthosis (TLSO) brace, the Boston brace is worn under the arm. This is why it is also called the "Underarm Brace" at times. The brace is created especially for a person with scoliosis with taking the body curvatures into consideration. The plastic is molded according to the body shape and there are three pressure points that are applied to help prevent progression of the curve. This brace is recommended for those who have a curve in the lumbar or thoraco-lumbar area and needs to be worn at least 23 hours in a day.

- *The Milwaukee Brace* — This brace, also called the Cervico-Thoraco-Lumbo-Sacral-Orthosis brace is similar to the Boston Brace but has a neck ring with vertical bars that attaches to the rest of the brace. It is prescribed for curves in the thoracic part of the spine and needs to be worn 23 hours a day.

- *The Charleston Brace* — The Charleston Bending Brace is sometimes called the 'night-time' brace since it is prescribed to be worn only at night. The brace is fabricated when the patient is bending to one side so that when the patient is in his normal position, the brace puts pressure in the opposite direction. This brace is effective only when the curve is below the shoulder blade

- *The Wilmington Brace* — This brace is also custom-made and is a total contact orthosis. It is created as a body jacket and can be opened in the front for easy removal. The corrective molds are fabricated in the body jacket to treat specific curves.

- *The Providence Brace* — This brace is made from an acrylic frame and applies corrective forces on the patient's body. Plaster impressions are taken in order to ensure that the pressure points used are exactly as they should be.

- *The Cheneau Brace* — Developed by Dr. Cheneau, this brace corrects the thoracic hypokyphosis. It is made from polypropylene and has a Velcro opening in the front. This brace aims at correcting the scoliosis in a three dimensional manner.

- *The SpineCor Brace* — This is a flexible brace that is prescribed for idiopathic scoliosis patients having mild scoliosis that ranges within curve levels of 15 degrees to 50 degrees. The patient is expected to wear the brace for at least 20 hours in a day. When the brace is made, it is expected that the patient will grow and therefore the brace accommodates this aspect. The parts of the brace need to be changed approximately every year and a half to two years. It has been seen that this kind of brace is extremely effective in juvenile idiopathic scoliosis patients.

While you may feel that bracing is an option that is non-invasive and therefore can be attempted, you should know that bracing does not really help in neuromuscular scoliosis or congenital scoliosis. It is also known to be less effective for infantile, juvenile and adolescent scoliosis.

Using a brace can be extremely embarrassing for some and it may also affect the self-image, especially among teenagers. Some go through a lot of discomfort on wearing a brace all throughout the day. This is why this decision should be taken after a lot of thought and consideration.

A study conducted on scoliosis braces in 1984 stated that braces do cause a slight, albeit insignificant, improvement in people who have been braced. However, there were observations that showed that 75 percent of the control group was also non progressive in nature. Therefore, assuming that the progression of the scoliosis curve can be captured and restricted may not be as clear as we may want to believe. The US Preventive Services Task Force stated in 1993 that "Beyond temporary correction of curves, there is inadequate evidence that braces limit the natural progression of the disease".

Drs. Dolan and Weinstein did a study in 2007 that was published in Spine. This study stated that mere observation and even the use of bracing did not bear an impact on the condition. Neither of these treatment options was effective in ensuring that surgery could be prevented. Ogilvie et al. at Axial Bio-Tech performed a study in which they studied the progression of the scoliosis curve and other related aspects among patients who were braced in comparison to the expected outcome of other patients based on the genetic knowledge. This study also showed that bracing did not have much effect on scoliosis.

The Spine Journal (September 2001) contained an article that was titled "Effectiveness of Bracing Male Patients with Idiopathic Scoliosis". This article detailed the manner in which a progression of 6 degrees was seen among 74 percent of the subjects despite the bracing. In addition 46 percent of the subjects using a brace reached a curve level that required surgery.

The Children's Research Center in Dublin, Ireland also published an article wherein it stated "Since 1991 bracing has not been recommended for children with AIS (Adolescent Idiopathic Scoliosis) at the center. It cannot be said to provide meaningful advantage to the patient or the community".

On the other hand, there are also some studies that have shown how bracing can be effective in reducing the progression of a curve at times. According to a study conducted by Scoliosis Research Society (SRS), bracing was successful in halting the progression of the curve in 74 percent to 93 percent of female patients with idiopathic scoliosis. The exact percentage of success depended upon the kind of brace used.

Despite various studies that have been done, there is still no definite answer to the question about whether a brace can stop progression or not. Matthew B. Dobbs, M.D., a pediatric orthopedic surgeon at St. Louis Children's Hospital and a study collaborator at Washington University states, "Even though bracing, to slow down curve progression in patients with AIS, has been the standard of care in the United States for about 30 years, the effectiveness of this treatment remains unclear. There are patients who use bracing, yet their curve progression continues. While on other hand, there are patients with AIS who do not use bracing without experiencing any curve progression." The Washington University School of Medicine in St. Louis is participating in a study to understand the manner in which braces affect different types of curves. It is expected that the study will yield answers and provide an insight into the specific type of curves in which braces is more likely to be successful. Researchers and medical professionals also believe that this will help in more selective prescription of a brace.

Research till date has not been able to unequivocally conclude that bracing is an effective treatment option for scoliosis. Dr. Stefano Negrini of the Italian Scientific Spine Institute of Milan, Italy reported along with his colleagues that there is no conclusive evidence of the effectiveness of the bracing option. The little research that does show that bracing is effective is also not conclusive in its findings.

Most of the people in the field of scoliosis treatment are awaiting the five year multi-million dollar study that is being conducted by National Institute of Arthritis and Musculoskeletal and Skin Diseases. It is expected that if this study is analyzed objectively, impartially and accurately, it will answer many questions concerning the effect of bracing and other treatments on scoliosis.

Based on the available information that we have currently, we cannot conclude whether bracing is an effective option or not. At least research has not been able to show conclusively that wearing a brace can improve the level of curve, reduce the amount of progression, prevent surgery or definitely help in any manner. There are so many factors that affect the manner in which the scoliosis progresses that there is little evidence to indicate that the few cases where bracing helped were indeed due to the bracing and not due to other genetic, nutritional, physiotherapy and environmental factors.

There are various drawbacks of wearing a conventional brace. For one, these braces are extremely uncomfortable. They are also very obvious and therefore are a definite "no-no" among teenage girls. The brace obviously needs to cover the chest area of the person completely. This is something that makes the body look bulky and gives a fair amount of discomfort to the person wearing it. In addition, most doctors who prescribe bracing also suggest that the brace be worn for at least 23 hours a day for it to be effective. There is little respite from the claustrophobic brace.

No doctor is ever likely to say this but the pressure that the brace puts on the body restricts mobility and movement in the natural way. It can also weaken the trunk over time and lead to muscle atrophy. The body becomes so used to wearing the brace all the time that the spine loses its natural power and strength. It becomes less flexible and can get injured easily when the brace is taken off. The constant pressure on the rib-cage can cause deformity of the chest leading to a higher level of complications in scoliosis.

We have also discussed about the psychological aspects of using a brace for scoliosis correction. Imagine being in a cast for the entire day and night. It is worse than living in armor because the armor can at least be taken off after a few hours and is not something that clings and puts pressure on your body all the time. A study conducted recently showed that 60 percent of the people in braces felt that they had been handicapped because of the bracing Fourteen percent felt that the bracing was a psychological scar. Would you want to do this to yourself or your child? It is an option that will probably be offered at some point in time and it might just help to review these objective points before deciding to put yourself or your child in a brace.

Another aspect that supports the fact that bracing is not effective is the lack of decline in surgical procedures that have taken place for scoliosis. Bracing is used by most conventional doctors in order to treat scoliosis patients. There are about 30,000 spinal surgeries that are done each year. Approximately a third of them are scoliosis surgeries performed for severe scoliosis cases. These cases do not seem to have reduced in number and are continued to be offered as the only option in the case of severe scoliosis.

While it is a good idea to be aware of the various pros and cons of bracing, there are some studies that prove their efficacy. In absence of any other form of treatment, this is the one therapy that one tends to resort to. Irrespective of what you decide after speaking to your practitioner, do make sure that you make the decision after being aware of all the pros and cons of using a brace, especially if this this an option being suggested for a teenager.

Types of Scoliosis Surgeries

There are also various kinds of surgical procedures performed in severe scoliosis cases.

Harrington Procedure

The Harrington Procedure was the most common of all techniques used in scoliosis surgery. However, this has been replaced with newer surgical procedures over the last 10 years. In this procedure, a steel rod is used that is extended from the bottom of the curve to the top. This helped in fusion of the vertebrae at the place where the correction was required. There were pegs too that were inserted in the bones. These acted as anchors for the rods that were suspended.

Post-surgery care involved the use of a brace to keep the posture in the right place for proper healing and complete bed rest for about three to six months. In most cases the rod could be removed after a few years once the correction has happened. But this was something that was generally not done unless there was an infection that needed attention.

There were some glaring disadvantages of this technique. For one, this procedure was extremely difficult to handle for teens. The three to six month complete bed rest could halt the life for a considerable period of time. There was some evidence of correction ranging from 10 percent to 25 percent in most cases but the procedure could not correct the rotation of the spine. This means that the rib hump could not be corrected. Most of the people who went through this procedure

Cross section of vertebra after scoliosis surgery

Screws are installed in the pedicles of the spine, and titanium rods ¼ inch in diameter are threaded through the heads of the screws.

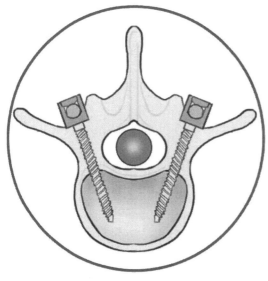
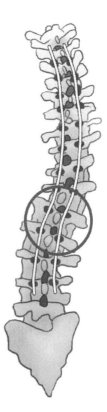

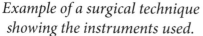
*Example of a surgical technique
showing the instruments used.*

ended up with a flat back syndrome. This was mainly because the correction removed the natural inward curving of the lower back called lordosis. Over time this syndrome started causing issues in standing erect later. If you have developed a flat back syndrome during this surgery, it might also cause an additional back pain during pregnancy. The Harrington Procedure was also fraught with issues concerning the crankshaft phenomenon. This s a condition that occurs when a part of the spine continues to grow after the partial fusion from back resulting in development of a curvature, since it twists the partially-fused spinal column. While this may not occur in those who are older, there is a higher chance of it occurring among children under the age of 11 years.

Cotrel-Dubousset Procedure

This surgical procedure is considered to be better than the Harrington procedure. It is thought to be effective in correcting the curve and the rotation of the spine and therefore is a step ahead of the Harrington procedure. The chances of a flat back syndrome are also extremely low with this technique. Parallel rods are cross linked to provide better stability to the fused vertebrae and the recovery time is about three weeks.

The biggest disadvantage of the procedure is that the surgery is extremely complicated and difficult to perform. There are too many cross links involved and the trained professionals who are adept at performing such a surgery with no complications are minimal.

The Texas Scottish-Rite Hospital (TSRH) Instrumentation

The TSRH procedure is similar to the Cotrel-Dubousset procedure to a large extent. The main difference is in the kind of rods and hooks that are used. They are smoother and better textured in the TSRH surgery. The texture and quality of the rods and hooks help in removing them later or readjusting them in case such a decision needs to be made a few months after the process. The disadvantages of this process are the same as those mentioned for the Cotrel-Dubousset procedure.

Luque Instrumentation

This is another procedure that surgeons have used for scoliosis surgery. This is a process that can help maintain the inward curve of the lower back. This process was thought to be good enough to obviate the need for braces post surgery. However, it was seen that without the use of braces, the amount of correction that was achieved after surgery reduced over time. The Wisconsin Segmental Spine Instrumentation (WSSI) is also a process that is used in some cases, but it seems to have all the negatives associated with the Luque and the Harrington Procedure as well.

Thoracoplasty is another procedure that has become extremely popular these days. However, this is a procedure that is likely to reduce the rib hump that occurs so often in the case of scoliosis. Sometimes this process is conducted along with spinal fusion. The surgery is fraught with pain in the ribs after the surgery has been performed. In addition there is also a huge risk of the pulmonary function being reduced. When this procedure is performed along with spinal fusion, it can increase the time taken to complete the surgery. This will mean higher levels of blood loss and prolonged anesthesia. It has also been seen that this is a surgery that can sometimes result in the puncture of the pleura. This can lead blood or air to drain into the chest cavity.

Typically, surgeons have used the posterior approach and the incision for the surgery has been made on the back of the patient. However, these days there is a tendency to use the anterior approach where the surgical opening is made through the chest wall. This is an option that reduces the chances of a crankshaft phenomenon in comparison to the posterior approach. The anterior approach is also better for correcting curves in the thoracolumbar region. The posterior approach is performed especially in cases when the sagittal curve needs to be decreased (in cases of hyper-kyphosis) and if there is a higher chance of infection to the lungs or chest.

There is no procedure that can guarantee 100 percent success when it comes to matters of health. However, when we give in to procedures that are invasive we give in to many complications that can occur. Studies done between 1993 and 2002 showed that scoliosis surgeries led to complications in 15 percent of children and 25 percent of adults.

There is a fair amount of blood loss that takes place during the surgery. This means that a large amount of blood transfusion is necessary during the procedure. Many patients are asked to donate blood during the pre-surgery period in order to compensate for loss; something that can be extremely stressful if one is already worried about the procedure and the outcome. Endoscopic minimally-invasive techniques are being studied in order to decrease blood-loss during surgeries.

As is the case with all surgical procedures, the opening up of the body increases the chances of infection. Urinary tract infections and those related to the pancreas are most common. Extended antibiotic coverage is essential post-surgery in order to ensure that the infection is prevented.

One of the largest complications of a spinal surgery is neural complication. These are known to occur among 1 percent of the patients who undergo surgery. Older patients are at a much higher risk of this complication than younger patients. Some of the outcomes of neural damage include muscle weakness and paralysis.

Pseudoarthrosis is a complication of scoliosis surgery in which the fusion does not heal well. This leads to a pseudo-joint developing in the spine. It is more common in the anterior approach and is known to have an incidence of 20 percent. The condition can be extremely painful and impossible to manage. The low back pain in such a condition is excruciating and can lead to disc degeneration over time. Over time, this affects muscle strength, mobility of the lower body and balance.

About two months after the surgery a significant percentage of young adults and kids have been seen to have pulmonary issues. This is a complication that has been seen in those who have secondary scoliosis. Other issues that surround the surgical correction of the scoliosis curve include gallstones, pancreatitis, intestinal blockages and other internal injuries that can occur due to dislodged hooks, breakage or rusting.

Over time, these surgical procedures have been reinvented and improved to include options that allow growing rods, vertebral body stapling and anterior spinal tethering. Many surgical procedures also claim to be minimally invasive.

The complications of a scoliosis surgical procedure are just too many to ignore. In addition, there is also the high cost of surgery to consider. The cost of this procedure in the United States is about $120,000 per operation. Slightly less than half the patients that undergo surgery seem to become disabled despite the surgery (or maybe due to it) and the remaining seems to go back to the preoperative stage within a maximum of 22 years. While the initial amount of the surgery itself is staggering, one also needs to keep in mind that there can be, and often are follow up procedures that need to be funded as well. Complications like loosening of rods, breaking of hooks and more may need to be repaired and in most cases require additional surgical procedures.

Can you imagine that about a quarter of those who undergo surgery seem to have issues with motor control after the surgery has been completed? There are many who actually go to the extent of stating that the complications that follow a scoliosis surgery are far higher and more difficult to manage than the scoliosis itself.

With consideration of these facts, one obviously does not wish to suggest that anyone go through this option in order to treat scoliosis. It does not even make sense when one will have a higher level of complications post-surgery and revert to the pre-surgical stage after some time. Yes, there are many surgical procedures that claim to be invasive to the minimum extent. But there is no real definition of minimally invasive. Also, when the body is opened for any kind of surgical procedure irrespective of how small the aperture is or how tiny the opening is, the chances of one complication or another increases. One can even think of taking such a risk when you know that the surgical process shall be able to correct the condition completely. However, this is not the case in a scoliosis surgery.

Choosing a technique that can help you manage your scoliosis better is an option that you have. Not only will it help you in the overall management of the condition it will also ensure that you are not taking high levels of drugs that are likely to make your system rot. If you want to correct your scoliosis to some extent before you conceive then think carefully before you choose surgery as an option. It is an option that will only lead to a weakening of your system; something that you do not want when you are preparing to host a baby inside you.

Surgery will require you to be bedridden for a long time before you can even think of getting up. This is not something you can do a year before you plan a baby. What this means is that, considering a surgical correction before thinking of getting pregnant is not a great idea. Not only can it lead to complications that can spoil your chances of bearing a baby in the next few years, it can cause complications that may affect your life.

After having read all the details about the complications of surgery and the high risks involved in addition to the lack of surety of the correction, do remember that in case your child is diagnosed with scoliosis later in life, you should make an informed decision regarding surgery as an option for him or her. In fact, make a note and refer to the various nutrition and exercise therapies that you can use in order to prevent the onset and progression of scoliosis. Remember what you have read about bracing. It is most likely not something you would want to go through and it is not something that you should choose for your child as it is a rigorous and debilitating treatment option.

There are various other methods that do not incorporate drugs, bracing or surgery and yet have been known to help in resolving the issues concerned with scoliosis. The Schroth method of physiotherapy has shown some success. It has been in use since 1920 and was developed in Germany by someone who suffered from scoliosis herself - Katharina Schroth. It is claimed that this set of exercises that was developed into a program have been able to help scoliosis curves by 10 percent. In addition to physiotherapy it is also essential that those who have scoliosis that inhibits normal work should undergo occupational therapy. This is normally the case with severe scoliosis. If you have a severe case of scoliosis and feel you are not able to manage your life, you must contact an occupational therapist to understand how they can help you. There is likely to be an assessment, intervention and therapy that follow the diagnosis.

Musculoskeletal Disorders reported a study in September 2004 conducted by Mark Morningstar, D.C., Dennis Woggon, D.C., and Gary Lawrence, D.C. In the study, 22 patients with a Cobb's angle of between 15 and 52 degrees were studied. These subjects were given rehabilitation protocols that included adjustments, exercise, vibratory stimulation and more. Out of the 19 people who completed the study, there was an average reduction of 62 percent and not any one of the patients showed any increase in the curve. Clearly, the study shows that there are ways and means by which scoliosis can be managed safely with therapy, exercise and rehabilitation.

As a would-be parent, you need to realize that the choices you make shall affect your baby in many ways. Therefore, you need to make sure that you manage and treat your scoliosis in such a manner that it is natural and without any risk to your system.

The one thing we know for sure about scoliosis is that it is hereditary. James W. Ogilvie's group has discovered genetic markers, two major genetic loci and 12 minor loci that can help us understand the development and progression of scoliosis. This means that hereditary predisposition towards scoliosis and the manner in which it is likely to progress is known. Since we know this, we can use customized regimens for treating this condition.

Most of the times, the conventional methods do not work because they attack the symptom and not the cause of the condition. This is the case with all medical treatment options that do not treat the individual but instead treat the curve only. It is important that any treatment be customized to the biochemical, neurological and metabolic factors that make up a human system as demonstrated in my first book, 'Your Plan for Natural Scoliosis Prevention and Treatment'. An effective treatment cannot be one that is common across all patients. A proper treatment that will bear results is one in which individual curve specification, lifestyle issues, nutrition and various other factors are taken into account to create a custom holistic treatment that involves diet, exercise and lifestyle modifications so that you are able to treat the condition and not just the symptom.

When you go to a doctor, they are trained to know what to give you and in all likelihood if your mother, brother or friend went to that doctor with the same symptoms, he would end up with the same prescription. Most of the drugs you consume will help you feel better because they reduce the severity of the symptoms. This is true for all kinds of ailments from flu, fever, common cold and headaches to heart disease and scoliosis. When you treat the symptoms and suppress them, you are telling your body that you want to ignore the signals that it is giving you. This is because symptoms are nothing but a manner in which the body communicates with you and tells you that there is something wrong that needs to be attended to. If you use the "quick fix" approach and "kill the messenger" you are not likely to solve the issues completely.

The view that most people have concerning the health of the body is uni-dimensional. They look at symptoms and then move ahead to look at ways and means by which they can be suppressed. This is merely a biological approach to the whole thing.

On the other hand, what is needed is a more holistic approach in which the practitioner understands the patient completely. This would mean understanding the fundamental imbalances that exist in the body and try to remove the imbalance completely. This book is designed to do just that for you. It is intended to help those women, who have scoliosis, progress through a healthy pregnancy without the need for drugs or surgical options before getting pregnant.

CHAPTER 7

PREPARING FOR A HEALTHY PREGNANCY

With scoliosis or without, preparing for a pregnancy is a task that requires extreme responsibility. You are deciding to bring another life into this world and it is your responsibility to do all that is in your power to ensure that the child is healthy. In addition, you owe it to yourself to take certain measures in order to ensure that your pregnancy is safe and uneventful to the maximum extent possible.

It is important to plan well before your pregnancy. Doing so can ensure that the entire nine months and beyond are set up for success. The planning is also important because a large number of the baby's organs start forming in the first few weeks. This means that your baby will start developing even before you know that you are pregnant. If you plan your pregnancy, you are likely to have an easier conception period, reduce the complications that generally arise during the early stages. You will also be able to recover more quickly from the delivery process and also minimize the risk of your baby getting any kind of health problem, including scoliosis.

Ninety percent of the couples who try to conceive do so in a matter of 12 months. Therefore, it is important that you give up all your vices and prepare to welcome a new human being into the world. At the same time, if it takes a while longer to conceive, do not listen to the various myths that surround pregnancy and scoliosis. Getting pregnant is not a switch that you can turn on and off; there is no magic pill that you can pop to help you conceive. The process is likely to take its own natural progression and time and it is best to use the known principles of counting the ovulation date rather than resorting to some surgical procedure or taking pills.

Most of the pills that you might take are likely to increase only the chemical levels in your body leading to issues later. Surgical procedures are not only expensive, but they can also leave your body weak and incapable of managing the pregnancy efficiently. In addition, there are no procedures that can guarantee that you will conceive – neither in the case of people who do not have scoliosis nor in the case of those who do.

Before you start to understand what you should do in order to try to increase your chances of conception, you need to know how fertility works. Katie Singer, who has been teaching Fertility Awareness since 1997, has arrived at various steps to follow in order to increase chances of conception. In fact, she states that it has been found that if done properly, the temperature charting method is as effective as the hormonal treatments, and that too without any of the side effects.

It is important that you understand fertility before you try to use various methods to enhance it. A woman's body moves through cycles of cooling and heating just like mother Earth. The levels of dryness and moisture determine the level of fertility that a woman has. If you are having a WOW moment while reading this, you have just discovered how the fertility of land and the fertility of a woman are linked. If you know the manner in which your body works, you may get to know the times when you are most fertile. Waking temperature, cervical fluid and changes to the cervix can be observed in order to take the guess-work out of the situation.

It might surprise you to know that the total number of eggs that a woman can ever produce is decided by the time a fetus is four months old. There are numerous follicles in the ovary, that house the eggs that have not been matured. At the start of a menstrual period, about a dozen of these follicles release estrogen. This causes a heightened increase in sex, the preparation of the uterus and the opening of the cervix. The body also cools down at this stage. Therefore, the signs of ovulation include a drop in temperature while vaginal fluid fluctuations are signs of a fertile time.

It is also important to know that a mature egg lasts in the outer edge of the fallopian tube for about a day or two. Depending upon whether you had an intercourse or not, or whether the cervical fluid in your body has been able to keep the sperm alive, the egg shall be fertilized or not. After this, the follicles start to produce progesterone that dries up the cervical fluid and warms up the body. The cervix also closes at this stage and a new uterine wall begins preparing if there has been no fertilization.

One of the most common reasons for delayed conception is the level of fat the body contains. The level of fat that you have can govern the ease with which you can get pregnant. The level of fat in the body should be within a certain range. Too much fat or too little fat in a woman's body can lead to issues with fertility. In some cases, this can actually cause the reproductive system to stop completely causing infertility issues. Fertility clinic data shows that about 12 percent of the infertility cases can be solved merely by managing weight and reaching the optimal level of body fat required for a healthy pregnancy.

The amount of body fat in your system affects whether you can conceive easily or not because the body requires estrogen, a hormone that is critical for the reproductive process. This hormone is stored in the fat tissues in the body. Lower levels of fat mean that the body does not have adequate levels of estrogen and higher levels of fat indicate that the body stores too much estrogen; more than what is required.

You can manage your weight issues on your own if you want to ensure that you conceive easily. The Body Mass Index (BMI) is a good measure that can tell whether you are overweight, underweight or are having the optimal weight for your height required for conception. The BMI is a tool that can be used to arrive at the weight status of all those who are above the age of 20 years. The various categories of BMI for women include:

- Underweight — Below 18.5

- Normal — 18.5 to 24.9

- Overweight — 25 to 29.9

- Obese — 30.0 and above

You can easily calculate your Body Mass Index if you know your weight and height. The formula for calculating BMI is weight / height squared. This is the formula that you can use if you know your weight in kilograms and height in meters. However, you will need to make some adjustments if you are calculating BMI based on the English system using pounds and inches as the units.

English BMI Formula

Weight in pounds / [(height in inches) x (height in inches)] x 703

Metric BMI Formula

Weight in kilograms / [(height in meters) x (height in meters)]

Why Gain Weight

Some women dread the thought of gaining weight. It's important to realize that normal weight gain during a pregnancy is not laying down as much maternal fat stores as one may think. The following table points out how those important extra pounds are distributed.

Breakdown of Your Weight Gain (All weights are approximate)		
Baby	7.5 lbs	3.4 kg
Placenta	1.5 lbs	0.7 kg
Amniotic Fluid	1.75 lbs	0.8 kg
Uterus	2.0 lbs	0.9 kg
Breast Tissue	1.0 lb	0.40 kg
Increase in Maternal Blood Volume	2.75 lbs	1.25 kg
Fluids in Maternal Tissues	3.0 lbs	1.35 kg
Maternal Fat Stores	7.0 lbs	3.2 kg
Total Average	26.5 lbs	12.0 kg

Once you know the Body Mass Index, you can see for yourself whether you fall in the underweight, overweight or obese category. In case you do not fall in the normal BMI segment and are having issues, chances are that your issues with fertility are related to weight. It is extremely common for people who have scoliosis to tend towards being overweight due to lack of exercise. Those who have not been managing their condition in consultation with a chiropractor may realize that they have slowly put on weight without really realizing the situation. There are also some cases that end up being overweight due to a sense of depression because they have scoliosis.

Then there are some people who become extremely concerned about their condition and consciously reduce the amount of food that they eat. In such cases, falling into the underweight category is common.

However, if you have identified the segment that you fall in, you can do something to increase or decrease the weight so that you can get it up to the optimum level. It is also important that you get the right amount of fat in your body because many nutrients that you will need throughout the pregnancy are stored in fat cells.

There is no reason for you to be too conscious of what you eat in order to avoid weight gain. This is the time to relax a bit and let yourself go. Start eating wholesome food that will help you add some good fat to your system. Monitor yourself regularly so that you do not overshoot your target.

If you are overweight or obese, you are likely to have high levels of estrogen in your body. High levels of this hormone act as the body's natural birth control because women who are overweight and do manage to conceive tend to have much higher chances of miscarriage.

A special note needs to be mentioned here concerning your partner's weight as well. Men who are underweight or overweight also tend to have a lower sperm count. You may want to ensure that your partner is not under or over weight in order to aid in successful conception.

Many people who have scoliosis feel that they should get a scoliosis surgery done before they start to think about pregnancy. While the surgical procedures may affect some of the symptoms of scoliosis and alleviate them, it is unlikely that the scoliosis will get cured forever.

And if you do decide to go in for a surgical correction, you will need to wait for at least six months to a year before you even try having a baby.

The Cleveland Clinic Journal of Medicine once stated that taking oral contraceptives is a useful method in which regular menstruation can be established especially with women who have Polycystic Ovarian Syndrome (PCOS). The fact is that oral contraception suppresses various kinds of functions that are part of the natural process of maturation of follicles, ripening of the eggs, emission of estrogen and more. The sad part is that the bleeding that does take place when you go off the pill is a kind of 'withdrawal bleeding' and not the shedding off the uterus lining as it is in the case of women who are otherwise healthy.

Of course, there are doctors who prescribe oral contraceptives as a method of birth control despite knowing about the effects it has on the body. The atrocity of it all gets even more bizarre when you think of the various drugs that are administered for the purpose of increasing fertility. Fertility drugs stimulate the ovaries and a larger number of follicles mature in comparison to the normal physiology of the body. This means that the level of estrogen that is produced is about four times more than the levels that are achieved on a regular or pre-drug basis.

An excess of these hormones can be extremely dangerous for the woman and the child that is born through such means. There are side effects and contraindications listed for the drug but the print is indeed so fine that you would require a magnifying lens to read them. The package insert that comes along with some of the fertility drugs is made available to the consumer only when they specifically ask for it. The reason is simple - the pharmaceutical companies are expected to state by law that the maximum number of cycles that the drugs should be used is limited to three or four times. That is clearly not what the manufacturers would want the consumers to aware of. There are women who have taken these fertility drugs for more than 12 cycles without knowing of the harm they are doing to themselves.

However, you can boost your fertility in various natural ways. If you feel that conception is taking more time than you thought due to your scoliosis condition, you can use some of the well-known holistic methods that have helped others in conceiving. These methods do not use drugs, chemicals or any kind of invasive methods that can harm your body in any way.

It is possible that if you are too worried about your scoliosis and the kind of pregnancy that you will have you may have difficulty in conceiving. Anxiety is closely related to infertility and issues with conception. Too much stress and worry can alter the chemicals in your body. Depression can also disturb the chemical balance in your system and keep you from conceiving. These are some controls that nature has already put in place. When you worry excessively about something or fall into depression, you are obviously not fit to take care of a new human being in the world. Nature tries to avoid a situation where someone who is unfit to take care of a baby should conceive.

When you are trying to conceive, try to keep your worries at bay. Read this book from start to finish and allay your fears about going through the entire pregnancy term with scoliosis. Make a trip to your gynecologist and your chiropractor and ask all the questions that may be popping up in your mind. RELAX and let yourself go! The more you think about it, the more difficult it will be to conceive. If you are taking any anxiety medication or antidepressants, you must stop doing so immediately. While there are some physicians who will tell you that it is normal to take these medicines when you are trying to get pregnant, remember that your baby already starts to develop before you can detect that you have already conceived. Risks of these medicines like benzodiazepines include birth defects, perinatal symptoms, behavioral disorders, hypothermia, deficiencies of muscle tone and more. The methods that you use to reduce anxiety or depression should be completely natural.

You can use meditation techniques to relax yourself. In addition, make sure that you surround yourself with positive people who do not raise your anxiety levels by talking about controversial and negative events. If you stay in the company of people who are positive, you shall be able to remain calm. Join a forum of women who have gone through pregnancy with scoliosis and you will be able to share your concerns with them. If you have the chance to meet women who have gone through the process without any issues, your confidence will increase and you will feel better and more relaxed about the whole process of conception and pregnancy.

Even if it takes a higher amount of time than you expected to conceive, do not let these worries enter your mind. Remain relaxed, count the days and try again! You need to give it at least 12 months before you start to take any active measures with regard to your conception if your weight is normal. Remember that scoliosis has nothing to do with the speed with which you conceive.

If you have been under the impression that positions during sex are only a matter of change, fun and to keep things interesting between the spouses, then you may be in for a surprise. There are some positions that are not as well suited for conception as others. For example, the woman on top position requires the sperm to travel against gravity towards the egg. This is obviously not the best position to have sex in when you are trying to conceive. The missionary position with the man on top is the best position to use when you are trying to conceive. It is also important that you lie in bed after you have finished up with your intercourse. Allow the sperm adequate time to travel towards the egg. Do not be in a hurry to get up and wash. In fact, prop a pillow under your hips to aid the path of the sperm towards the egg.

There are other very basic aspects of being able to conceive that you may want to know. These are based on observations over the years. The viscosity level of your cervical mucus decides the rate of travel of the sperm towards the egg. The higher the fluidity of your cervical mucus, the easier it is for the sperm to travel through it. You can take some herbs that are known to help in increasing the cervical mucus. These include ashwagandha, shatavari, yashtimadhu, ashoka and kumari. You can also keep a track of your cervical fluid by checking the toilet paper every morning. The quality of the fluid changes based on your menstrual cycle. It moves from sticky and glue-like to milky in consistency to slippery and watery like an egg-white. The latter is the best and most fertile mucus that can help sperms to survive for longer periods in the body by providing the required nutrients.

Green leafy vegetables and fresh fruit juices are known to nourish the reproductive system. Even when you are trying to conceive, it is not recommended that you go at it like rabbits. Restraint from frequent intercourse may help your partner produce healthy and resilient sperm that can travel all the way up to the uterus before giving up!

Make sure that your partner is also doing his part in the attempt to make a baby. If your partner smokes, make sure that he stops the habit and gives up on any illegal drugs that he may be taking. Wearing boxers is relatively better than wearing briefs; loose fitted pants are better than tight jeans. This ensures that the testicles are cooler while they are placed away from the body so that they can produce more sperms. Many oriental cultures believed that the man also needed to consume a nutrient rich diet in order to conceive and they were right in assuming so.

Liver, red pepper, carrot, oatmeal and apricot contains adequate vitamin A that helps in increasing sperm count. Heidi Murkoff mentions in her popular book 'What to Expect When you are Expecting' about how vitamin A deficiency is linked to a sluggish sperm count and therefore reduced male fertility. Other foods that can help you increase vitamin A levels naturally are lettuce, spinach, sweet potatoes and broccoli. Vitamin C also affects sperm motility and viability. The antioxidants that are contained in asparagus, snow peas, cooked tomatoes and strawberries may also help in increasing the sperm count.

Men can end up with low testosterone levels due to low levels of zinc or lead. This is also something that can reduce sperm count. High levels of folate are not important only for women but also for men since low levels can produce a larger number of chromosomal abnormalities.

Do not consider the process of making a baby a chore. It is something that you need to enjoy with your partner despite the calculations and planning. So dress up for him and do something unusual because women who enjoy their partners are known to be better sperm receivers.

Try making out in the dark in order to reduce the production of melanin, a hormone that can regulate other reproductive hormones. This can sometimes affect your menstrual cycle to aid conception.

Along with your mind, your body also needs to be ready for the baby. This means that you need to prepare a healthy ground that will receive the baby. While there are some things that you need to avoid, there are some that you need to include in your lifestyle to become ready. A large part of this relates to the diet that you have and the level of activity that you include every day. Here are some of the things that you need to include and exclude from your diet and activities when you are preparing for pregnancy.

Things to Include

1. *Multivitamins* — It is a good idea to start taking a multivitamin when you decide that you will start trying for a baby. It is important that you receive these vitamins from natural and whole foods so that you maximize the amount that is absorbed. When the body recognizes the natural foods that you consume, it begins to absorb the vitamins contained in the foods far more efficiently than when you take them in form of concentrated pills. Conventional vitamins and supplements are chemical isolates do not have wholesomeness and benefits of natural supplements.

2. *Folate* — Folic acid has been known to promote neural development in the fetus.

3. *Fat* — Relatively larger levels of fat are required in the body for the preparation of a pregnancy. This is however, essential when you are not otherwise overweight. Full fat dairy products are known to improve fertility. It is advisable that you use some butter to flavor your food instead of using margarine or vegetable oils. Other healthy options for fat include olive oil and coconut oil.

4. *Protein* — Adequate levels of protein can start preparing your body for the times when you will need all the protein that you can get for the baby. At this stage of development, protein is a

critical nutrient that you need to provide for your baby. Fish, beans and eggs are a great source of protein during pregnancy.

5. *Cod Liver Oil* — This is one ingredient that both traditional and oriental societies have believed in. Folklore says that fish oil was used in cases where there were fertility issues. Recent studies have also shown that cod liver oil helps in increasing fertility fluids, ensuring healthier pregnancies and producing richer and healthier breast milk too.

6. *Zinc* — Zinc is known to be great for women who have scoliosis. It is also an element that your partner may want to increase in his diet. Zinc contributes significantly to male fertility. One of the best sources of zinc is shellfish.

7. *Fluids* — Top up on the fluids but do make sure that they are the right ones. Consume a lot of water, soups, herbal teas, milk and your body shall stay non-toxic and clean.

Things to Avoid

1. *Caffeine* — Caffeine has been associated with endometriosis; the presence of endometrium that causes premenstrual pain and dysmenorrhea. This is something that your partner should also give up in order to ensure that their sperm is healthy.

2. *Alcohol* — While a single drink once in a while may not impair your abilities to conceive, it has been seen that moderate levels of alcohol can impede estrogen production. A study showed that if you reduce the amount of alcohol that you consume to less than five drinks per week the chances of conception can increase significantly.

3. *Nicotine* — This is a complete no-no. Smoking is known to destroy eggs and in case you conceive with one of these eggs that have been damaged by the nicotine levels in your body, you may have a child with some congenital disorder. If you are a smoker, then quit now and stay away even from second hand smoke for at last three months before you start to think of conceiving.

4. *Drugs* — This does not refer to hard street drugs that all of us know are harmful for the body. It refers to any medication that you may be taking. If you are taking any kind of medication for any condition, you must discuss this with your gynecologist and make sure that it is safe for the baby that you are planning to conceive.

After having done all this, if you are still having trouble conceiving, there are some specific steps that you can take in order to make sure that the sperm gets to the egg when the ovulation takes place. This might make you feel that you are being calculative about it, but you will need to take some specific steps towards conception. There are some signs that will tell you when you are almost ready for ovulation or have just ovulated so you know when it is the right time to have a go at it.

You can use a special thermometer to measure your basal body temperature. These special thermometers can help you monitor small changes in temperature. Keep a diary in which you note the temperature daily. Your temperature is likely to be lower than normal in the few days preceding ovulation. Once you ovulate, your body temperature will start to rise and stay there for some time before it starts to drop again before the next cycle. Make sure that you take the temperature at the same time every day so that the diurnal variations in temperature do not alter the readings.

The cervical fluid is another thing that you can monitor to know when you are about to ovulate. Take a tissue and wipe the vaginal area to check the cervical fluid. As you approach ovulation, the fluid becomes milkier and creamier and then move to being slippery like an egg white. This is the time when you are about to ovulate.

Head to the bed when you notice signs that tell you that ovulation has occurred. These are the best days to ensure that you conceive. As you start doing these things to ensure higher chances of getting pregnant, make sure that you follow the diet mentioned above, get your weight to a normal range and exercise enough to improve the circulation to your reproductive organs. Starting a pre-natal yoga routine can also help your body prepare for the baby. It also relaxes you so that you can enjoy the process of getting pregnant rather than making it a chore.

Going to a fertility clinic or to a doctor is not the first thing you should do if you are not getting pregnant, In fact you should keep in mind that most people take about a year to get pregnant and therefore make the decision of visiting a fertility clinic only after you have tried everything and continued with the above mentioned practices for at least one year. Conceiving naturally is possible for you and your scoliosis condition does not prevent conception. Do not worry if it is taking some time to get impregnated.

If you do have to see a fertility doctor, then get some basic fertility tests done. This will include a sperm count for your partner. Ask for the non-invasive tests that you can use initially before jumping in and trying everything that you can.

Last but not the least you need to make sure that you are emotionally and financially prepared for the baby. These are basics that you need to think about when you bring a baby into this world. You should be in a position to give a lot of time, love, care and comfort as well.

CHAPTER 8

NOW THAT YOU ARE PREGNANT — THE FIRST TRIMESTER

Realizing that you are pregnant can be a time of great joy. There are things that you will look forward to and the anticipation of the arrival of a new life in the house fills everyone with joy. Make sure that you enjoy this time and feeling to the fullest.

There are many signs of pregnancy that you should be aware of. These are signs that will get you thinking in that direction so you can get a pregnancy test done at home or at the clinic to officially confirm your beliefs. Here are some signs of early pregnancy to keep a look out for.

- *Amenorrhea* — This is the most common sign of pregnancy and refers to the absence of a menstrual period. Sometimes a menstrual period can be missed due to excess travel, fatigue, hormonal disorders, extreme weight loss or going off the pill.

- *Morning sickness* — This is a feeling of nausea that may or may not be accompanied by vomiting. While it is called morning sickness, it can occur at any time of the day. Women can develop morning sickness at any time between two to eight weeks of being pregnant. Nausea can also be caused by food poisoning, emotional stress or other illnesses.

- *Frequent urination* — Something that can start as early as two to three weeks after conception, frequent urination is another sign of pregnancy. It can occur due to diabetes, stress or a urinary tract infection as well.

- *Tingling or swollen breasts* — The breasts start to change almost as soon as conception occurs.

Some of the other signs of pregnancy that you may notice in the first trimester include darkening of the areola or the dark area around the nipples, blue and pink lines under the skin on the breasts and food cravings.

Most people confirm that they are pregnant with the use of a home urine test. This is a simple kit that you can use to affirm whether you are pregnant or not. The kit indicates the result that can be understood from the self-explanatory note. The home kit detects the presence of the hormone hCG (human chorionic gonadotropin) in the urine. The results of a home test are mostly accurate but if you do get a positive it is recommended that you go to a lab and get a pregnancy test done for confirmation. The only negative of the home test kit is that if you are pregnant and the kit inaccurately shows a negative, your first visit to the doctor may get delayed. A medical examination confirms the pregnancy without any doubt. This physical examination is likely to include the uterus examination, which is likely to be enlarged, or cervical examination which is likely to be soft and have a different texture.

With pregnancy, there comes great responsibility. You feel that you need to do all the right things so that you do not hurt the fetus in anyway. It is also a fact that your body is undergoing many changes. In fact by the time you realize that you are pregnant, you are already likely to be a few weeks into the pregnancy.

There are a lot of things that you will need to do but before you start to understand the specifics, it is important that you also understand the changes that your body is going through and what you can expect from the various doctor appointments that you will now have to go for.

Good prenatal care is an extremely important part of pregnancy. Therefore, make sure that you choose your doctor well. Make sure that you choose someone that you have extreme faith in so that you will feel at ease discussing every aspect of your pregnancy with him or her. In addition, you should ensure that you tell your gynecologist about your scoliosis condition so that he/she is aware of what to take care of. It is, in fact, a good thing to introduce your gynecologist to your chiropractor or the physician who is treating you for scoliosis so that they can compare notes and arrive at the best option for you in terms of nutrition, exercises and prenatal care.

While it may seem like it is too early, you should try to discuss the various kinds of delivery options that you have so that you can start preparing for it. Consider having birthing rooms, birthing chairs, water birth and home birth. The concept of a Leboyer bath is also something that is catching on where childbirth is ensured into temperature-controlled water, without being harsh on the newborn child. The lights in the delivery room are dimmed so that it is easy to make the transition from the dark uterus to the light of the world. Slapping the baby on the bum is also something that is not recommended in this kind of birth. The umbilical cord is kept intact until the baby and mother get to know each other for the first time and it is cut off only after a while.

Screening

Now that you are pregnant, considering your health history becomes extremely important. Some of the things that you may need to think about include previous pregnancies or abortions, general health, diet, fitness levels and history of multiple caesarian operations. You should also check whether the child has the same rhesus blood group as you or not. Different rhesus can cause issues during the delivery process and so you need to be aware of it. If you have had any history of fibroids, endometriosis or incompetent cervix, you will need to remain in the constant care of a gynecologist.

The screening for Down's syndrome is done in the first trimester of the pregnancy. The screening involves an ultrasound to check excess amounts of fluid behind the fetal neck. A blood test is also done to check levels of plasma protein A and hCG. This screening is done between the 10th and 14th week of the pregnancy. Other screening tests that you could consider include CVS (Chorionic Villus Sampling) that is known to be able to detect more than 3800 disorders that are related to the gene pool. However, this test requires you to give a sample of the placental cells via the vagina.

Changes in Your Body

The first trimester is where you will start coming to terms with the fact that you are pregnant. While it may not be overt, you may still experience certain symptoms that point towards pregnancy. Some of the things that you feel physically include high levels of fatigue and sleepiness, frequent urination, nausea, vomiting, heartburn and indigestion, food cravings and aversions and changes in the breasts. Emotionally you are likely to be relatively unstable with mood swings and irritability.

As you enter the second month, you are likely to feel some amount of weight gain. The weighing scales will start showing it too. Frequent urination, nausea, food aversions and cravings and fatigue are likely to continue. You may start getting a whitish vaginal discharge and slight headaches. Some women also experience weakness and giddiness. If you are feeling weak, you may want to ensure that you take care of this aspect and do not rise suddenly from seated position. You may also start to notice your clothes getting tighter around the abdomen.

The third month has similar symptoms but you may actually start getting your appetite back and may realize that you feel like eating more. This is also the time when you slowly become completely at peace with the fact that you are pregnant and accept the changes that are happening to your body. A sudden calm and tranquility is what you are likely to feel as well.

Making it More Comfortable at Work

If you are a working person, then it is necessary that you make sure you are comfortable at work. Make sure that you take time for three well-balanced meals a day. Your breakfast should be relaxed and hearty. The saying that breakfast is the most important meal of the day has an increased importance and significance during pregnancy. Keep a few healthy snacks in your work area so that you do not find yourself hungry or working late without anything to nibble on.

Despite the frequent urination that you are experiencing, drink at least 64 ounces of water every day. If you feel that going to the water cooler every now and then is an issue, get a nice handy bottle and carry it along during meetings as well. Comfortable pregnancy clothing is readily available easily these days. So as soon as you feel that your skirt or trousers are becoming tight, invest in some maternity clothing and ensure that you do not wear tight clothes to work. Staying uncomfortable all day may not be the right thing to do.

Do not stay in the sitting or standing position for too long. This will become even more important as you progress in your pregnancy and therefore requires specific note. If your work involves standing for long periods of time you may want to invest in a small stool that you can put one foot on to relieve the stress on your back. If you have a desk job, taking frequent breaks to fill up your water bottle or going to the washroom may ease off the pressure. Use a comfortable chair to sit and work in. If you do not have a particularly comfortable chair, speak to your superior and check if you can get one that is ergonomically designed to relieve the pressure in your lower back. While this is something that is beneficial for all moms who are pregnant, it is particularly important for you due to your scoliosis condition. Take time off to make your working area comfortable.

Avoid lifting heavy objects and stay away from areas that are smoke-filled. Carry a toothbrush with you to work to clean your teeth after every meal and if you are suffering from morning sickness then carrying some mint and candies may ease the nausea.

Make use of some of your casual leave options and take a day off simply to relax and chill out. Carry headphones to work and listen to relaxing music when you are not doing something that needs all your attention. Listening to music can also be extremely relaxing and good for the baby.

Make sure you listen carefully to your body. If you feel particularly tired on a specific day, call it quits early and offer to do your work from home or check your mails from home if you have the ability and strength.

Miscarriage

The possibility of miscarriage is highest during the first three months. Many people do not announce their pregnancy to the world in order to keep it a private affair till the time that they are over this difficult period. There are various factors that can cause a miscarriage and there is a lot to be learnt about the specific factors that cause it. Of a higher level of concern are however, the myths that are associated with miscarriage. You can rest assured that miscarriages are definitely NOT caused by previous trouble with IUD, history of multiple abortions, temporary emotional stress, skeletal conditions like scoliosis, minor falls or injury, sexual intercourse or physical activity that one is accustomed to.

The factors, that we do know, which can increase the chances of a miscarriage include poor nutrition, smoking, hormonal insufficiency, bacterial infections, congenital heart diseases, kidney disorders, diabetes and thyroid infections. It is important that you are aware of these aspects so you can ensure that you take extra precautions. However, do not worry about an occasional cramp, ache or a little bit of spotting.

Some of the possible signs of miscarriage include severe cramps in the center of the lower abdomen or bleeding. A sign of concern is if the pain does not stop for a long period time like a full day. Light staining for three days continuously or heavy bleeding should be brought to the notice of the gynecologist immediately.

Managing Stress

Do not let stress about the pregnancy or anything else affect your state of mind. It can cause sleeplessness, depression or anxiety, none of which is good for your health or your child. Stress also causes you to become negligent towards your pregnancy and result in lack of appetite or binging on the wrong foods.

If you are disturbed about something it is a good idea to talk about it. Make sure that you continue to communicate with your spouse about what you are going through. This is especially necessary if your partner is not reading upon the changes that are happening in your body, on his own. He needs to understand the level of complications and changes that you are going through in your life so that he can adjust and participate in them too. Other people you can talk to about your situation or concerns are your family members, a friend, your gynecologist or someone else you trust.

Sit back and think of the reasons why you are experiencing stress. A large part of the battle against stress can be won if you are able to identify the cause of stress. This means that you will be able to do something about it. Sleep off your stress if you have to and make sure that you use relaxation techniques to stay calm. If you feel that a specific situation is causing you too much stress, then get rid of the situation permanently.

Heartburn and Indigestion

With the pressure that the curved spine puts on the various parts of your body due to the scoliosis along with a growing uterus, heartburn and indigestion are very common. The first thing that you need to know is that while you struggle with your heartburn and indigestion, your baby is completely oblivious to the trauma that you are facing in this area. Just make sure that you do not let this situation influence the nutritious diet that you are supposed to consume during this period.

One of the main reasons you may be experiencing heartburn is the tendency that all of us have to overindulge in food when we are pregnant. Other than that, there are also specific medical conditions that may cause your heartburn. Early in the pregnancy, the high levels of progesterone and relaxin produced by the body tend to relax the smooth muscles in the gastrointestinal tract, allowing the food to move upwards into the esophagus, thereby causing heartburn and a feeling of bloating.

If you are dreaming of a miracle that will relieve you of heartburn completely, then you should know that it is impossible to have a pregnancy without going through this. In fact, the slowdown of the digestion process that is caused helps the intestinal tract to absorb a large amount of nutrients from the food you eat in a more efficient manner.

However, this does not mean that you cannot do anything to reduce the symptoms of heartburn or try to prevent it from happening too often. While you should eat healthy, try not to gain too much weight. Large amounts of weight causes more pressure on the stomach and therefore may make it tougher to deal with heartburn. It is a good idea to ensure that the weight gain per trimester is within the normal range. This should be a total of 25 to 35 pounds from the time of conception to the day of delivery. You should gain between 1 and 4.5 pounds in the first trimester and between 1 and 2 pounds every week in the second and third trimesters. Eat smaller meals in a day but eat more frequently. This allows the food to get digested before you put some more in. Do not gobble your food in a hurry. Take your time to chew and swallow it. Try to identify specific foods that give you heartburn and eliminate them from your diet.

Do not wear clothes that are tight around the abdomen and remain upright after a meal for at least a few hours. Prop yourself on a pillow while sleeping. This is something that will help as you move into your other trimesters as well. If the symptoms are too much to bear, look for some alternative or natural gastrointestinal tract relaxant.

Constipation

Another issue that is extremely common among pregnant women during the first trimester is constipation. The hormones that have caused your muscles to relax also lead to sluggish muscles in the lower abdomen causing difficulty with elimination of feces. While this is a normal phenomenon among many pregnant women, you can take some steps to relieve the situation.

Add large amounts of fiber to your diet and include fresh vegetables, fruits, cereals and dried fruits. Avoid any kind of canned or processed food. Not only does this kind of a diet help in relieving constipation, it is also extremely nutritious for you at this stage. Taking a large amount of fluids will help you fight back constipation in a very aggressive manner. Flush your system with lots of fluids and do not forget that water is extremely good for your health too.

Don't hold up an urge to defecate because you are busy with something else. Go to washroom when you have to. Check the supplements that you are taking. Some calcium and iron supplements cause constipation and you may want to discuss these with your practitioner in case you feel they are causing constipation. Exercising regularly can relieve you of this problem. However, given your condition of scoliosis make sure that you refer to the exercise regime detailed in the chapter later in this book so that you do the right exercise that can benefit you in your pregnancy and not cause any complications.

Weight Gain

Gaining extra weight during pregnancy, when you are also suffering from scoliosis as well, is easy. Exercise is not the first thing that is likely to come to your mind during pregnancy in any case with all that you are going through. And when you are riddled with the prospect of dealing with the scoliosis as well, it is not something that you may want to look forward to along with scoliosis. Excess weight gain is likely to cause additional issues with your condition and therefore should be avoided at all costs.

The important thing to note also is that any extra weight that you gain cannot be lost. You can also not adjust that weight gain in the next trimester because your baby needs a constant supply of nutrients to grow. So if you have gained extra weight in the first trimester, still you cannot hold yourself back in the second trimester in regards to nutritional intake. Just make sure that you are careful about eating right in the next trimester too.

Weight gain during pregnancy should be optimal. The amount of weight that you gain should be higher than 20 pounds. But excessive weight can cause issues too. Ideally the amount of weight that you gain should be between 20 pounds and 35 pounds. The rate of weight gain should be around 3 to 4 pounds in the first trimester, 12 to 14 pounds in the second trimester and 8 to 10 pounds in the third trimester.

Weekly Changes to Watch Out For in the First Trimester

The counting of weeks for pregnancy starts from week 4 with the first week counted from the day you started menstruating last time. This ensures that the dates are more accurate. Below is a summary of some of the changes that you will see in the various weeks to come in your first trimester of pregnancy.

- ☐ *Week 4* — You will obviously have a missed period that will hint you towards confirming your pregnancy. Nausea, vomiting, dizziness, headaches, bloating, feeling of fullness, appetite loss and frequent urination will be common. Some women may also experience light spotting due to implantation. Your baby will still be an embryo and about 1/25 of an inch in size, and is therefore not likely to put any pressure on your spine as yet.

- ☐ *Week 5* — Fatigue will usually set in by the fifth week. There will also be hormonal changes that may begin to make you feel more irritable and emotional. The breasts are also likely to feel more tender. Sleeping in a sports bra may help. In most cases, morning sickness will start at this stage, if it has not been already set in. You may also start getting used to getting up for urination every now and then.

- ☐ *Week 6* — The symptoms that presents so far are likely to get more pronounced in this week as the body works hard to prepare for the baby. Craving for specific type of food and aversion towards some of them may start. Make sure that you start eating healthy food and in adequate quantities, even if are experiencing a loss in appetite. The baby is likely to be around 0.2 inches from the crown to the rump but he or she is likely to be curled up making specific measurement still tough at this stage.

- ☐ *Week 7* — In addition to the initial symptoms, you may also start experiencing some constipation, vaginal discharge and excessive salivation. Feeling dizzy or light-headed and bouts of indigestion may also be common. This is also the stage when your abdomen will start to expand and tight fitted clothes may become difficult to wear. Start investing in some maternity clothes to help ease your day.

☐ *Week 8* — The uterus will be about the size of an apple at this stage. Fatigue, swollen breasts, acne and slow digestion shall continue. The slow digestion causes bloating but it also helps in better absorption of the food that you consume so that you can assimilate the most of what you are eating. It is advisable to have small but frequent meals and avoid fatty foods.

☐ *Week 9* — A stuffy nose and heartburn are likely new symptoms that may add on to the already long list of symptoms that will be facing. Mood swings are extremely common and you may find yourself crying at the drop of a hat. Warn your spouse about this so that he is not taken aback by your changed personality.

☐ *Week 10* — Changes in complexion are likely to begin at this stage. You may notice blotchiness and acne and the weight gain will also be likely to start showing. Specific care shall be taken of oral care since pregnancy gingivitis is a common complaint that many women may have.

☐ *Week 11* — This is the time when the uterus will start enlarging just above the edge of the pubic bone. This means that very soon enlargement of your abdomen will start getting visible too. You should maintain good posture so that you do not have frequent complaints of back pain.

☐ *Week 12* — The last week of your first trimester will herald the initiation of pregnancy glow on your face, giving you something to feel good about. A higher level of blood volume and increased oil gland secretion brings about a plumper and smoother skin. This is also the time when you will start seeing the morning sickness vanish in most cases. Even though you will be becoming heavier, fatigue will vanish.

CHAPTER 9

CARRYING THE WEIGHT: THE SECOND TRIMESTER

The arrival of the second trimester brings a sigh of relief for most pregnant women because it is supposed to be the easiest of the three trimesters that you will go through. However, for a person with scoliosis it brings some challenges as well. While you will feel a reduction in the various symptoms that you witnessed in the first trimester, there will be new challenges that you need to face as the baby grows inside you.

By this time your uterus will be about the size of a small melon. The baby inside you will also be about five inches and will weigh about the same number of ounces. The body starts to grow at a faster rate than the head and therefore the proportions of the baby start to resemble human proportions in this trimester. By the time you reach the end of the second trimester, your baby should have reached about 12 inches in size and about two pounds in weight. At this stage your baby will start to move and press against the uterine wall too. Even though the vocal cords are developed, the baby does not speak in the uterus. Fetal hiccups, however, are common and should be something that you will face off and on.

Changes in the Body

The symptoms that you have been experiencing in the last three months are not likely to disappear immediately as the second trimester starts. You may still experience some amount of fatigue and tiredness and occasional headaches. Indigestion is also likely to continue. As you gain weight you may also start experiencing some swelling in the ankles and varicose veins. By the fifth or sixth month, leg cramps may start too.

The difficulty in carrying the child becomes tougher as the abdominal area becomes larger. You may start experiencing higher levels of back pain as you progress. It is recommended that you do not take pain killers to ease off the pain that may be higher than normal due to your scoliosis. Use alternate methods of relieving pain and discomfort and continue to do the exercises that have been listed.

You may also experience some whitish vaginal discharge. This discharge is likely to increase as the second trimester proceeds. These are a normal part of pregnancy that you need not worry about. By the end of the fourth month you will also start feeling some movement in the fetus. This can be a great source of joy as you feel your baby move inside you and respond to your voice. However, it is also likely to make you jump from time to time as he pushes in certain sensitive areas.

The movement that you may feel in the fetus can be experienced like a twitch, butterflies in the stomach, a growling feeling or sometimes even as if someone has socked you in the stomach. This depends on the specific kind of movement that the baby does.

Working Till the Last Day

Many women think that it is best to continue working until the last day of the pregnancy because it gives them the opportunity to spend their entire maternity leave with their child. While this is something that you can definitely do, you need to think about a few things before you make that decision. The most important aspect of this decision is something that your own body can tell you. It has been established that there is no harm in working until the end, even if you have a strenuous job. This is because women who have jobs that require them to stand most of the time also have bodies that are used to that kind of strain and exercise. Listen to your body and if you feel that you need some rest, take your maternity leave a few days before the due date.

A certain amount of breathlessness is common among pregnant women who reach the second trimester. While the hormones are to blame for the continuous feeling of short breaths, this is mild enough not to disturb your daily routine, but could hold you back from strenuous activities. On the other hand, if you experience severe breathlessness and your extremities start turning blue, you need to see your practitioner immediately.

Sleeplessness

With the excitement, stress and anxiety that pregnancy brings and a belly that is growing at a fast pace, catching up on sleep can become extremely tough at times. While these sleepless nights may give you a feel of the sleepless nights that you will experience once the baby arrives, you do need to get plenty of good sleep to allow the baby to grow adequately.

Getting a good amount of exercise can also help you feel tired enough to sleep. Good exercise does not mean a power schedule that can be harmful for your body but one that can relax you adequately and prepare your body for delivery. Some great exercises include stretches, yoga and kegel exercises.

Despite the fatigue that you may be feeling, try to avoid taking a nap in the middle of the day. This does not mean that you should not take rest breaks and lie down for a while during the day. Instead catch up on some television in a comfortable position or read a pregnancy book to prepare for the arrival of your child.

Make sure that you create a bedtime routine that you start identifying with sleep. This should start with a dinner that is consumed leisurely. Do not gobble up your dinner. A dinner with the family is a great idea but if you cannot ensure that, you can sit and have a slow, leisurely and relaxed meal. Do not have a heavy meal before sleeping and make sure that you have a few hours between supper and bed-time. Follow the routine with a warm bath or light reading and use some aromas that can make you feel even more relaxed.

Maintain a good environment in the room that you are sleeping in. Make sure that there is no ambient noise and that the air conditioning is neither too cold nor too warm. Keep the lights off and make sure that you do not associate the bed with anything else except sleeping. Reading in bed or watching television while you are lying down may take you away from the sleep. Using a comfortable mattress is also extremely essential. Prop and fluff the pillows so that you have a good backrest to avoid heartburn if it is one of the symptoms that is keeping you from sleeping.

While drinking a lot of water is a good thing, frequent need to go to the washroom at night can keep you awake for a long time. Try to limit fluid intake after 6pm to reduce your night trips to the washroom.

If you are someone who is used to sleeping on the stomach, sleeping while you are pregnant may be extremely tough. It is a traumatic situation because you are never truly comfortable at least like you are used to. In fact, sleeping on the back is also not a recommended position for you since it is likely to put a lot of pressure on your lower back causing back pain. The best position for sleeping is lying on your side. You can cross one leg over the other and place a pillow between the legs for maximum comfort.

Backache

In addition to the scoliosis condition, your body is undergoing many changes that can cause backaches. The joints of the pelvic area that are generally very stable start to loosen up in order to prepare a wider and easy passage for the baby. In addition, the over-sized abdomen can cause a lot of pain in the lower and upper back too. When you start to curve your shoulders back to regain the balance, you put a lot of pressure on the lower back causing excess strain.

Doing all that you can to prevent this kind of pain is the best option. The first thing that you need to understand is that excessive backache is not an option that you can be 'okay' with. You should ensure that you do everything in your power to gain the right amount of weight that you should have during the pregnancy. Do not flip over to the other side and reduce the amount of nutrition that you are supposed to consume. But yes, there is no doubt about the fact that gaining even an extra pound, beyond what you should ideally put on in terms of weight, is not a good thing for you.

Make sure that you maintain good posture and do not slouch as you work on the computer. Be careful about bending your back and make sure that you bend from your knees when you are lifting something off the ground. Abrupt movements are to be avoided at all times and try to use your arms for lifting rather than your back. Always sit comfortably in a chair that provides good lower back support. Get up every now and then because sitting in one position for a long time can also be something that can cause higher levels of backache.

Wearing high heels is not good when you are pregnant. Keep your stilettos and even moderate heels in the cupboard and make sure that they stay there for a while until you are back to your pre-pregnancy weight after delivery. If you are facing issues with a lot of weight, check with your doctor whether you can wear a pregnancy support sling.

Relief can be obtained from the backache by using alternate cold and hot press. Use an ice pack for about 15 minutes and then follow it by a hot towel for the next 15 minutes. Visiting a chiropractor or a physical therapist may be a good idea to relax the pain.

Low Lying Placenta

To make space for the baby to grow, the placenta also moves around your abdomen. It is estimated that about 20 to 30 percent of women have the placenta in the lower part of the abdomen in the second trimester. This condition is called placenta previa. However, there is no need to worry about this early on because the placenta continues to move and can move upwards in most of such cases.

Accept the Pain of Delivery and Prepare for it

Whether it is a delivery for someone who does not have scoliosis or for someone who does, the pain of delivery is something that a pregnant woman needs to accept and come to terms with. There are some women who prefer not to know anything beforehand about the pain that they are likely to suffer during the process. While this may keep them less anxious for some time, the fact is that they are not likely to be prepared for the various eventualities that may arise.

A better option is to prepare for what you are likely to go through and also experience the various eventualities that may arise during childbirth. This preparation involves making your mind and body ready for the process of delivery.

The first thing that you need to do is to get educated about the process of delivery. Not everyone has the time to go to education classes and if you are one of them, then reading up as much as you can will help immensely. Don't just read and stop there, do something about it. Make sure that you do the prenatal breathing exercises and the kegel exercises so that your body is far more flexible during the process.

While there is no denying the pain of childbirth, there are some very positive sides to the whole thing. For one, labor cannot go on forever and therefore you know that it will end. An average labor lasts from anywhere between 12 and 14 hours and only a few hours among these are really uncomfortable. The other thing is that there is a definite purpose for this pain and when you hold your baby in your arms, you are likely to forget about the trauma immediately. While you are going through the pain, losing sight of that purpose is very natural and not something for which you should hold yourself guilty.

Don't try to be the epitome of tolerance and decide to do it on your own. It is a good idea to have someone who will mop your brow, massage your back, feed you ice chips and keep you calm and breathing correctly.

Do not try to be a martyr by refusing pain relief completely. If this is something that you feel strongly about, then talk with your doctor and make your preferences known to the physician who is going to deliver your baby. Remember, this is not a test that you can pass or fail. You will not be awarded the best mother of the year if you deliver vaginally or without medication – there are so many methods to deliver your baby and your having scoliosis does not negate the various delivery options available.

Childbirth Class

There are various benefits of taking a childbirth class. There are many classes that will take into consideration your scoliotic condition and recommend the right exercises for you. Check with your chiropractor whether he has a specific class that he can recommend for you. In case you are not able to find a class that suits your exact needs, make sure that you learn these exercises from your scoliosis physician, so that you are doing the right thing for yourself and your baby.

A childbirth class helps you meet with other expecting parents and therefore provide you with an opportunity to discuss your apprehensions, excitement and progress with them. Given that they are in a similar phase in life, talking to them about your feelings will be far easier than talking to someone who has not been through pregnancy. Such classes also increase the involvement of the father in the process of pregnancy and childbirth. These classes help you in achieving a less stressful labor by preparing you physically and mentally with the use of breathing exercises, relaxation techniques and more.

Try to find forums online where you can speak to other women with scoliosis who have gone through childbirth so that you can hear their experiences. This will give you the much needed confidence at this stage about the fact that all will end up well and you only have to prepare for it.

A good childbirth class is one that is recommended by your practitioner and your scoliosis physician. If you can find one specifically meant for pregnant women with scoliosis, it would be ideal. A class should not have more than five to six expecting parents and it should include discussions on various kinds of delivery options, medication during delivery, actual breathing and relaxation techniques and question and answer sessions.

Weekly Changes to Watch Out For in the Second Trimester

The second trimester is considered to be relatively easier than the first one. However, for those of you who have to manage scoliosis and pregnancy at the same time, there are some specific changes that you need to look out for. Some changes that you will see in this trimester are:

☐ *Week 13* — As the risk of miscarriage reduces with the start of the second trimester, anxiety levels shall reduce. You are also likely to get used to your pregnancy by now. However, this is also the time when the uterus will start growing and you may feel some abdominal pain as the ligaments stretch to accommodate the growing uterus. The baby is likely to be about 3 inches long. The baby can also move his or her legs and arms but it is too early for you to start feeling the kick as yet.

☐ *Week 14* — With higher levels of energy you may be tempted to do more work than usual. Remember that it is best to listen to your body carefully and not exert yourself to hurt your lower back in any way. Add fiber to your diet to help manage constipation. Some of the previous food cravings may be replaced with new ones at this stage.

☐ *Week 15* — Lower levels of immunity are likely to make you more susceptible to common illnesses. It is a good idea to be extra vigilant about hygiene at this stage.

☐ *Week 16* — Some women start to feel 'quickening' or the first movements of the baby. These are more like the flutter of a butterfly in the stomach rather than the kicks that we hear about so often. Almost 5 inches now, the baby will start to put higher levels of pressure on your spine.

☐ *Week 17* — Most women start to feel the baby move at this stage. Increase in appetite is also common at this stage. Make sure that you consume a healthy diet (detailed in chapter 11) that is fit for pregnant women with scoliosis so that you can address both things at the same time.

☐ *Week 18* — The uterus is the size of a cantaloupe at this stage. As your heart will start doing extra work of pumping blood into the fetus, feeling of dizziness and light-headedness by you will get common.

☐ *Week 19* — A more active baby who can turn, kick, twist, wiggle fingers and toes and move arms starts to bring on some challenges to backache management. This is not something that is a large cause of concern among women who do not have scoliosis. However, you need to be extra careful about backaches and the damage an added pressure on the spine can cause.

☐ *Week 20* — Not only is there a pressure on your spine but the pressure on your lungs may cause short breaths. Pressure that the uterus puts on the urinary bladder will compel you to go to the washroom more frequently than before. Make sure that you visit the washroom regularly and do not try to rush at the last minute; something that may cause accidents.

☐ *Week 21* — The center of gravity of your body is likely to change as the belly grows larger. Make sure that you give up all jerky movements and get up or sit down slowly. It is essential that you gain the right amount of weight while continuing to eat healthy. Discuss this with your doctor to monitor the amount of weight that you will gain every month.

☐ *Week 22* — Some babies can be as tall as 10 inches at this stage and as your uterus rises above your navel you may also see some stretch marks on your belly.

☐ *Week 23* — Some of the symptoms of the third trimester start to appear towards this stage. Braxton Hicks contractions, heartburn, leg cramps and general discomfort with the larger belly may be things that you may have to deal with.

☐ *Week 24* — At this stage you could have put on about 20 to 35 pounds. The movements of the baby are also likely to increase significantly.

☐ *Week 25* — The uterus is likely to put a lot of pressure on your back and pelvis. Issues with sciatica, or radiating lower limb pain, can also arise at this stage as the uterus puts pressure on some specific nerves. Pain in the lower back, legs and buttocks are likely to cause some trouble at this stage.

☐ *Week 26* — The last week of your second trimester, now is the time when Braxton Hicks appear in most women. These contractions are mild and similar to menstrual cramps. You may also experience some pain along the side of the abdomen like a stitch.

CHAPTER 10

THE LAST THREE MONTHS: THE THIRD TRIMESTER

With the start of the third trimester you start feeling that the end is closer than the beginning now. Many women continue to feel great in their last trimester. But there are also many for whom the stress starts to show. The backaches and other aches in the body start to show on your face and you feel that you are hardly looking like the glowing pregnant woman that you thought you would be. For many women this is a stage that they literally want to pass through in the blink of an eye.

Changes in the Body

At this stage, many women become so used to being pregnant that it does not matter anymore. In the third trimester you are likely to gain the maximum weight in the seventh and the eight month. The amount of weight gain is not so high in the last month, closer to delivery. Fetal movements are likely to be far stronger and more frequent at this stage. Constipation and heartburn may continue. Swelling in the ankles and varicose veins are extremely common in this trimester. You may also continue to experience shortness of breath and difficulty in sleeping with a large abdomen. Braxton Hicks contractions are also something that you may start experiencing in this trimester. These are small contractions that are almost always painless. Your breasts are also likely to become larger and heavier and some colostrum may also leak during the last month.

Emotionally, there is a lot that is likely to be going on in your mind. It is like a crescendo of all the feelings that you have had all this while. The excitement of the baby's arrival mixed with the prospect of suffering the pain of delivery causes emotions that you had never felt throughout pregnancy. You are likely to be bored of the pregnancy and may want it to end as soon as possible but make use of the most of this time in preparing for the arrival of the baby by designing the nursery or buying clothes because you are unlikely to have loads of time once the baby arrives.

Lower Back and Leg Pain

One of the many side effects of the joys of motherhood is pain in the lower back and legs. This is likely to be more exaggerated in your case due to the pre-existing scoliosis condition. The enlarged uterus is likely to put pressure on various nerves of the spine, the most common of the lot being the sciatica nerve. This causes a lot of pain in the lower back, the buttocks and the legs too. Applying cold and hot compresses alternately and resting adequately will help provide pain relief. Refer to the pelvic tilts mentioned in chapter 12. Visit your chiropractor, who may suggest some specific alternative and natural medication to relieve the pain, if it is too much to bear.

Abnormal Pulmonary Functions

Pregnant women with scoliosis can face serious breathing problems, especially during the final stages of pregnancy when the body exerts extraordinary pressure on the back to adjust the growing baby. In cases of women whose scoliosis is associated with a neuromuscular condition such as poliomyelitis or muscular dystrophy, a severely restricted lung size might create an abnormal pulmonary function or breathing problems. Refer to the box below to know more on how to measure the lung size.

How to measure lung size?

A simple blowing test is the best way to measure vital capacity to assess the lung size. This test can be used to measure the total amount of air which is actively expelled from the lungs after a person has taken his maximum breath. A specialist's review is recommended in cases where the vital capacity comes out to be 50% less than the expected level.

Sources :
- Simonds AK. Kyphosis and kyphoscoliosis. In Albert RK, Spiro SG, Jett JR, eds. Clinical respiratory medicine. New York: Mosby, 2004; pp 765-69.
- Shovin CL, Simonds AK, Hughes JMB. Pulmonary disease and cor pulmonale. In Oakley C, Warnes CA, eds. Heart disease and pregnancy. Oxford: Blackwell Publishing, 2007: pp 151-72.
- Shneerson JM, Non-invasive ventilation in pregnancy. In Non-invasive ventilation and weaning: principles and practice, Elliott M Nava S Schonhofer B, eds. London: Hodder Arnold, 2010; pp 496-98.

Research throws up interesting evidence with regards to the effect of the vital capacity on the level of complications a pregnant woman with scoliosis might face in her third trimester. Though lung size is a useful parameter, yet it has been seen that women with a vital capacity of around 0.8 litres can do well with respiratory support. In fact, the outcome is expected to be good as long as the capacity exceeds 1.25 litres.

However, a lung size below this capacity is sure to create problems, primarily characterized by a reduction in the oxygen levels or hypoxaemia. Generally, this stage of low oxygen levels can worsen during sleep and exercise and can bring along a increase in concentration of waste gas or carbon dioxide . The box below explains the concept of non-invasive ventilation, a helpful method to help pregnant women with scoliosis, suffering from low oxygen levels.

Non-invasive Ventilation

For the purposes of non-invasive ventilation, a small breathing machine can be used for pregnant women having low oxygen levels, especially those with a vital capacity of less than 1 litre or those having weak muscles. Proper use and regular monitoring of this machine can ensure successful results for both, the baby as well as the mother.

Apart from the lung size, hormones can also play a role. The three key hormones, namely, oestrogen, progesterone and relaxin undergo drastic changes in pregnancy. These hormones actually cause the ligaments of the pelvis and lower spine to loosen to facilitate an easy birth. In fact, the breathlessness seen in the early stages of pregnancy is partly caused by this rise in progesterone. It will stimulate breathing by increasing the respiratory rate and also the depth of every breath. Other physiological changes like an increase in blood volume might also happen.

Another important fact to know at this stage is that women diagnosed with adolescent scoliosis are usually not likely to have a low vital capacity. Regular breathing tests might be all that is required to check for the proper functioning of the lungs.

Heart Defects and Abnormalities

In certain cases, the early onset of scoliosis is related to a congenital heart defect, for instance, a hole in the heart. Though such issues are often spotted and rectified in the childhood, yet it is important to get an ECG and an echocardiogram of the heart done to rule out any potential complications. As long as the oxygen level of the mother and the heart function is as required, there should be no reason to worry.

Birthing Plan

Many people feel that working out a birthing plan helps them stay focused and move ahead with the last three months of pregnancy. There are some practitioners that have a ready format that their clients can fill out. Typically the plan includes the parent's preferences concerning the hospital for childbirth and the specific procedures that they would be fine with. It is not considered a contract of any sort but it is a manner in which the practitioner can understand what the parents would like the childbirth to be like.

The birthing plan includes the specific center where you want the birth to take place, the amount of time after labor begins that you would like to be at home, your choices for eating or drinking during labor, possibility of walking or sitting during labor, personalization of the atmosphere of the labor room conditions, use of a video camera during childbirth and the use of a mirror to view childbirth. The plan also details the preferences concerning procedures like delivery positions, use of oxytocin, use of pain medication and anesthetic drugs, and use of forceps or vacuum or caesarean. Making your desires known about holding the baby immediately after birth and feeding should also be made clear so that the authorities do not whisk your baby away before you have had a chance to meet your little one.

Pain Relief during Labor and Delivery

Irrespective of what people might say regarding scoliosis and labor, the prerogative of deciding whether you want pain relief during labor and delivery still belongs solely to you. There are various kinds of pain relief options that pregnant women can use. These include anesthetics that numb sensations, analgesics that ease the pain and ataraxics that tranquilize the patient.

The epidural block is the most common kind of medicine that is used during delivery. This option can be used for caesarean as well as vaginal deliveries. It is one of the most preferred options because it numbs the lower part of the body without the need for complete anesthesia with a minimal amount of dosage. Some people feel that the side effects of an epidural block include shivering, prolonged numbness and occasional headaches post-delivery. But these are far less common and few. As an alternate to the epidural block, a pudendal block can also be opted for. This is mainly used in the case of vaginal deliveries and is administered in the perineal or vaginal area. This option does not reduce the discomfort arising from the uterus but takes the pain away when forceps or vacuum need to be used.

The most common analgesic that is used for delivery pain is meperidine hydrochloride. It is delivered intravenously but may need to be given every three to four hours. The alternative medicine options available for labor and delivery are growing by the day. There are some women who choose hypnosis or TENS (Transcutaneous Electrical Nerve Stimulation). Acupuncture is also a very common alternative that many choose along with distraction, hydrotherapy or physical therapy. However, these therapies have not been researched too extensively. It would be a good idea to do your own research and then decide if you are comfortable with any of these options.

Presentation of the Baby

The manner in which the baby lies is something that your practitioner can tell you by palpating. The head is generally round and smooth and the other way to get an idea of the position is the location of the heartbeat.

The vortex or the head down position is the most common. This is the position that makes a vaginal delivery possible. A breech position is when the baby has the buttocks towards the vagina or the legs are facing downwards. If the baby is lying sideways, the position is called transverse.

The specific kind of delivery option available for you, if your baby is in a breech or transverse position, should be discussed with the gynecologist. There are no absolute causes of a breech position but it can be caused by a smaller than normal fetus or when there are more than one fetus. A breech position is also possible if the uterus is unusually shaped or has fibroids. Sometimes it may also be present when the amount of amniotic fluid is too much or too little.

Caesarean

A caesarean may not have been one of the popular delivery options some years back, but today it is a widely accepted option. In most cases, one cannot say for sure whether you will require a caesarean section or not. However, one should always be prepared for the eventuality. There are however, some cases where the doctor does not have any option other than a caesarean. These include instances where the mother has a specific infection of the uterine passage or the baby needs to be removed from the uterus immediately without any trauma. Placenta previa is also another situation where a caesarean becomes necessary. If your doctor perceives that a caesarean is necessary in your case due to any specific indication, you should discuss the specifics of the caesarean beforehand.

Having a caesarean section is an option that you should discuss with your practitioner towards the end of the eighth month. This is because your gynecologist will be able to tell you exactly about the condition of your uterine passage and whether you will require a caesarean section or whether you can try to go for a natural delivery.

Caesarean sections – Trend and Complications

Latest research definitely shows a higher incidence of caesarian sections in women with scoliosis, especially those who've had corrective surgery done. A study amongst 142 pregnant women who've undergone such surgeries revealed that the proportion of women who delivered with the C-section was slightly higher than the general population. However, the rate of complications was no higher. Though, around 40% of mothers did develop a low back pain during their pregnancy, yet it mostly resolved within the first three months, post delivery.

Source: Orvoman E, Hiilesmaa V, Poussa M, Snellman O, Tallroth K. Pregnancy and delivery in patients operated by Harrington method for idiopathic scoliosis. Eur Spine J 1997; 6:304-07.

In women considering caesarian section as option, it is important that the concerned obstetric anaesthetist be informed in time. This is important so that alternative ways to administer an epidural can be decided, especially in women who've had a corrective surgery done for scoliosis in the past.

It should be borne in mind that your scoliosis in no way rules out options of getting a natural vaginal delivery, but your specific case may need to be evaluated by your gynecologist.

Being Prepared

If you have not yet started thinking about what you will pack in your hospital bags, then the beginning of the ninth month is the time to do so. You need to make sure that you pack everything you may require in the hospital, so that your husband does not have to run at the end time to get items that you need. The bag with things that you will need for the baby shall be packed and ready to be picked up on the way out of the door when the time comes. Keeping your hospital bag in the car is also a good idea in case you are not at home when labor begins.

Try to make one bag for the baby and one for yourself so that things will be easy to find. Include copies of the birthing plan, a timer, a CD player, the video camera, a book to read, lotions and creams, a tennis ball for massage, a comfortable pillow, tooth-brush, tooth-paste, soap, heavy socks, slippers, nightwear, hairbrush, hair-clip and a few clothes. You need these because you can never be sure whether you will end up having a caesarean for which you may need to over-stay at the hospital for recovery.

For the baby's bag, include a sterilized bottle, clothes, wrap, blanket, sheets and a woolen cap for the head. Mittens and booties for the hands and feet are also a good idea. Make sure that you include diapers, wet tissues and a diaper rash cream along with baby soap and baby lotion.

Pre Labor and False Labor Signs

The anticipation that you are likely to feel by the time you are in the ninth month is quite high. This is because you probably start thinking of the time when the baby will arrive in your arms. You may find yourself thinking about labor and contractions all the time. But you do need to know that there are many women who experience false labor, get to the hospital or are midway towards the hospital only to realize that the contractions were not for real.

Contractions that are not regular or those that do not increase in frequency or intensity or contractions that subside when you start to walk or move are indicative of a false labor. A show that is brownish in color is not indicative of labor but more a sign of an internal exam or intercourse in the last 48 hours.

On the other hand there are some specific symptoms that will tell you that labor is approaching and that you need to start preparing, if there are some things that you need to complete, before heading off to the hospital. The sad part is that these symptoms can start to occur as early as a month before labor. And sometimes these may start to manifest themselves only a few hours before the labor starts.

About two to four weeks before labor, the fetus begins to move downwards into the pelvis. This is accompanied by an increase in pressure in the pelvic area and the rectum. You may also experience a persistent low back pain. A sudden downward trend in energy is also experienced by those who are close to labor. The vaginal discharge is also likely to increase in quantity and thickness. Braxton Hicks contractions become more frequent and the loss of your mucous plug is also common.

Real labor symptoms include contractions that are regular and those that intensify each time. A show or pinkish blood streak is also a sign that you are likely to get into labor. A membrane rupture and the process of the water breaking is a sure sign of the fact that you need to get to the hospital.

Weekly Changes to Watch Out For in the Third Trimester

The third trimester is especially trying for those who have scoliosis. This is mainly because of the ever increasing pressure that the uterus puts on the spine. But this is also the most challenging trimester for all mothers since the wait becomes too tough and you cannot wait to see your little one in your arms.

☐ *Week 27* — The pelvic muscles will start to strain at this stage and doing kegel exercises may help immensely. Your baby will have been formed completely by now weighing about 2 pounds or more. A large part of the brain development also happens at this time.

☐ *Week 28* — Your weight and the baby's weight are likely to continue growing larger. You would have become used to Braxton Hicks contraction by now. Sometimes the movements of the baby are likely to put additional pressure on your spine and this may cause additional discomfort too.

☐ *Week 29* — Your baby will require a lot of nutrients to ensure that the internal organs and the brain develop at a healthy pace. Even though energy levels may be down, try and continue your exercises like walking and swimming. Do some exercises that strengthen abdominal muscles supporting your back as well.

☐ *Week 30* — Constipation and heartburn will be the normal complaints at this stage. Foods high in fiber content can help in reducing constipation and smaller meals well before bedtime help in managing heartburn. Swollen ankles can be managed by ensuring that you keep your feet raised up and drinking loads of water.

☐ *Week 31* — Sleeping may become difficult with a large belly but try and get in as many winks as you can and avoid foods that keep you awake like caffeine.

☐ *Week 32* — Some issues that occur commonly in this stage include breathlessness and fluid retention. With the baby getting larger, he/she may not have much room to move around and therefore the kicks and punches may become less frequent.

☐ *Week 33* — From this time to delivery, your baby gains about half the birth weight and therefore you may see a lot of weight gain happening at this time. Your belly will also increase in size significantly.

☐ *Week 34* — Aches, pains and exhaustion reach an all new level at this stage. What you will need to concentrate upon at this time is that this is not going to last for too long.

☐ *Week 35* — Increased pressure on the veins, the rectum and the spine are what you will experience in this week. Hemorrhoids are also likely and you need to drink lots of fluids to be able to manage that.

☐ *Week 36* - This is the time when your baby is accumulating fat and becoming chubbier. You may also be asked to undergo an internal examination to check whether the cervical dilation has started yet.

☐ *Week 37* — At this stage, you pregnancy is almost full term. If labor starts at this stage, it will not be stopped and you will be allowed to deliver your baby. You can sit back and relax about any apprehensions that you may have had about a premature baby.

☐ *Week 38* — You should start reading about labor and the delivery options that you have. Discuss this with your doctor and decide the kind of delivery that you want.

☐ *Week 39* — You can start to get signs of labor any time now. Hang in there and wait for the labor to start.

☐ *Week 40* — By this time you will have already crossed your due date. The doctor will wait for a few days if you have not delivered already and then decide on a date for the delivery.

CHAPTER 11

THE PREGNANCY DIET TAILORED FOR SCOLIOSIS

The importance of diet during pregnancy cannot be emphasized enough. It is something that has become extremely important in the modern day times due to the kind of lifestyle that we have. Pigging out on junk food and living stressful lives is not something that is likely to be great for the baby or your own health.

The foods that we eat these days are highly processed and have no similarity to the kind of food that was consumed by our ancestors. While the technology has grown by leaps and bounds, allowing us to pack foods in various tetra packs, cans and vacuum sealed bags, the fact is that our body has not been able to evolve as quickly as the technology. This means that our body is not programmed to digest the processed food easily. The response is invariably an inflammatory one and something that is likely to cause your body to react negatively.

Evaluating what your ancestors ate can help us eat right and live healthy. This is something that applies not only to pregnant women but to anyone who wants to live healthy too. The story of Weston A. Price and his research into the Paleolithic diet are extremely interesting.

It was in 1930s that Weston A. Price, a dentist from Cleveland, started conducting some experiments to understand the reason for disease and degeneration among the modern population. He is often referred to as the "Albert Einstein of Nutrition" emphasizing the kind of depth in his research and the discoveries that he has found in the 10 years of his experimentation.

Price travelled globally to check out the health status of people who had not been influenced by modernism or western civilization in order to study the manner in which they had progressed in terms of health. As a dentist, his first observation was that dental caries, deformed teeth, crooked teeth and cavities were a result of the modern day diet that comprised of sugar-rich, candied, canned or processed food. It was established that these issues were not a result of bacteria, viruses, genetics or brushing habits.

His expedition that lasted for six years across all the continents of the world made him unearth various truths of life that many modern day nutritionists and doctors are not willing to believe. He studied the isolated villages of Switzerland, Gaelic communities in Outer Hebrides, indigenous people of South and North America, Melanesian and Polynesian South Sea Island people, African tribes, Australian Aborigines and the New Zealand Maori. The first observation was that the amount of whole grain and unprocessed food that these communities and tribes consumed was far higher than what we consume in today's world. This kind of food provides four times more water soluble vitamins and minerals and about ten times more fat soluble vitamins in comparison to the modern day diet. He also discovered a fat soluble nutrient that seemed to be missing in our modern day diet that was not known before. He decided to call it "Activator X".

Most of the communities that Price studied had strong built and the women had far easier reproduction and delivery as compared to the modern day situation where a large number of pregnant women end up on the caesarean table. He also found that the level of degenerative ailments like heart diseases, diabetes, cancers, etc were almost absent in the communities. Emotionally too, these people were more happy, more content and stress-free.

In fact, he was the one who found that the diet we consume is also responsible for the "borrowing" phenomenon that leads to the body borrowing nutrients from the skeletal system leading to a reduction in the size of the skeleton. In some cases this shrinkage has been reported to cause a loss of as much as 10 inches in height. This borrowing makes the bones weaker, thereby resulting in bones that are more prone to scoliosis and osteoporosis. It is also a fact that this phenomenon of borrowing tends to occur mostly among women because modern day society puts a lot of pressure on women to maintain ultra-thin figures. The bones get weaker and the spine curves, leading to various kinds of skeletal issues. This can cause many problems during delivery and lead to higher levels of back pain.

If you were to see some of the images presented in Dr. Price's classic volume, "Nutrition and Physical Degeneration", you will see the huge difference between handsome healthy people that are primitive and the stress-ridden emotional manifestations of degeneration in the modern population.

Based on his research, the Weston A. Price Foundation created a table of differences for the traditional and modern diet:

Traditional versus Modern Diets	
Traditional Diets	Modern Diets
Foods from fertile soil	Foods from soil depleted of all nutrients
Organ meat preferred over muscle meat	Muscle meat preferred. Organ meat almost negligent
Natural animal fat	Processed vegetable oils
Raw or fermented dairy products	Pasteurized or ultra-pasteurized dairy products
Soaked or fermented grains and legumes	Refined and extruded grains and legumes
Long fermentation soy products consumed in moderations	Industrially processed soy products consumed in large quantities

Traditional versus Modern Diets	
Use of broths	Use of artificial flavors and monosodium glutamate
Unrefined sweeteners like honey and sugarcane	Refined sweeteners
Lacto fermented vegetables	Processed and pasteurized vegetables
Lacto fermented beverages	Modern soft drinks
Unrefined salt	Refined salt
Natural vitamins that are found in food	Synthetic vitamins taken as supplements or added to food.
Traditional forms of cooking	Microwave cooking
Traditional seeds and open pollination	Hybrid and GMO seeds

Courtesy of The Weston A. Price Foundation

It is obvious from the above table that the food consumed by our ancestors has been changed. The United States of America has now taken it upon themselves to reduce the amount of obesity that they find in their country. They are now considering this as a national threat to the country where one in every ten residents is obese and one in every four people who enlist for the army recruitment is rejected due to obesity.

Clearly, processed food is one part of our modern day diets that should be avoided at all times when you are pregnant. They tend to be high in sugar, carbohydrate, fat content and salt and are very low in nutrients and therefore cause many issues that you simply will not like to face when you are going through your pregnancy neither will you like the complications that could arise.

- Processed food can cause obesity and are likely to make you put on more weight; something that you cannot afford due to your scoliosis condition.

- Processed food causes imbalance in digestion, leading to higher levels of complications concerning heartburn, indigestion and acidity.

- Processed food has also been linked to depression, memory loss and mood disturbances, an aspect that is already heightened during the pregnancy. The last thing that you would want to do is consume processed food and add to the havoc that the hormones are playing inside you.

- While these canned and packed foods are supposed to have labels that are accurate and precise, the fact is that the practices are far from perfect. Some labels will state that it is "sugar free" but may contain other forms of sweeteners like "agave" or high fructose corn syrup that are equally harmful.

- It has also been identified that the deficiency in vitamins caused by lack of easily dissolvable vitamins and minerals can lead to difficulty in conceiving and infertility too.

- Chemicals, pesticides and herbicides used in farms today, are also known to lead to scoliosis in animals. This is something that has been observed and is still under investigation. Kepone, a pesticide, is known to cause scoliosis in fish and pesticide exposure to tadpoles causes spinal curvatures as well.

- In addition, processed food has been linked to cancer too.

Most of the health issues that are arising among the modern population, concerning issues with natural processes, are due to the diet that we are all taking. Over the years, manufacturers of various kinds of foods have inculcated different myths in the market. The proponents of specific kinds of fad diets have also played a large role in popularizing them. While some expect you to cut out all carbohydrates from your diet to lose weight, others insist that any kind of saturated fat is a bad thing. Here are some of the beliefs about food and nutrition that have made their home in our minds that may actually not be true. Read through them and you will realize the number of fallacies that you may have in your mind concerning food and nutrition.

Saturated fats — If you thought that all kinds of saturated fat are something that you need to avoid for better overall health and particularly for the heart, then you may need to get some fundamentals right. A certain amount of saturated fat is essential for the body. It provides support to the cell walls and helps in the production of fatty acids. It also helps build immunity levels and makes your bones and lungs stronger. The amount of calories that you consume as fat should depend on the level of activity that you have and your metabolic type. It should definitely not be lower than 30 percent of all calories consumed in a day. Even the National Institute of Health (NIH) acknowledges that a certain amount of fat is required to absorb vitamin A, D, E and K. They are also important for children since they are required for their proper growth and development. Saturated fats provide the building blocks for cell membrane development and hormones. They are also essential for converting carotene into vitamin A. Contrary to general belief they also lower cholesterol levels (palmitic and stearic acid). It also acts like an antiviral agent to protect the body.

Cholesterol — Cholesterol has always been considered to be an evil thing that we need to get rid of. It is often stated that there are two kinds of cholesterol that we have in our body – LDL and HDL. The cholesterol theory that has been talked about for so long also states that LDL cholesterol is the bad cholesterol while HDL cholesterol is the good cholesterol. However, this entire theory started with the 'Lipid theory' that stated that cholesterol diets led to deposits on the arterial walls. Later, research showed that 80 to 90 percent of the cholesterol in the body is actually produced by the body itself, proving that the diet plays an insignificant part in cholesterol formation. Even the study popularly called the 'Seven Countries Study' is flawed with issues. The study proved that the countries having a national diet that was high in cholesterol had a high correlation of deaths caused due to heart diseases. However, what was not questioned was why the data from the remaining 16 countries not considered for the analysis. This is a classic case of using data to lie statistically.

Red meat — The development of the nervous system is also enhanced by the consumption of red meat that consists of various nutrients like vitamin B12, vitamin B6, zinc, carnitine, phosphorus and co-enzyme-Q10.

Eggs — Another food that helps in the nervous system development is eggs. With the advent of egg substitutes, the consumption of this great protein of nature has been limited.

Grain — While many think that some amount of grain is required by the human body, what needs to be remembered is that man was a meat eater. The nutrient-rich diet provided the nourishment required to survive the winter months. Even after farming started, the grain used was partially germinated and sprouted since it used to lie stacked in the fields leading to fermentation due to rain and mist. Refined flour does not have any nutrients and you will only be adding empty calories to your system by consuming white refined flour.

Modern Day Pregnancy Diet Suggestions

The amount of advice that you will start receiving as soon as it becomes evident that you are pregnant is something that can be difficult to digest. Some people will tell you about the foods that you should not consume because they are harmful for your health and the baby's health and others will tell you about the specific kinds of food that you should eat. Be thankful if you have not been given a menu that you should follow. While all these suggestions are likely to have good intentions, they only tend to increase the paranoia of someone who has recently discovered that she is pregnant.

One could say that perusing books on pregnancy can help in eating well throughout the nine months to ensure that you provide adequate nutrition to the baby. Unfortunately, it is not as simple as you might think.

You need to walk down the aisle of bookstores that are labeled "baby and childbirth" or "pregnancy" and you will realize that there are too many books to choose from. Some of them are written by doctors while others are compiled by obstetricians, midwives, nutritionists and even other pregnant women. The sad part is that most of the books are surprisingly similar in nature and use the food pyramid as a guide to suggest the foods that you should be eating.

The fact remains that none of these books seem to have done any research on their own and seem to be regurgitating any other advice that could come their way. Just because the same thoughts are written by many people does not mean that it is to be believed blindly. In fact, some of the recommendations that have been presented in these modern day books are incorrect and may actually keep you away from some of the great foods that you should be consuming during this phase of life. Some of the suggestions that they have made in comparison to what Weston A. Price had found in his study are discussed below.

- *Seafood* — There is one aspect of the modern day pregnancy books that is right. The fact is that fish contains high levels of Omega-3 fatty acid that is extremely good for health. Omega-3 is an anti-oxidant and it has various other qualities that can keep you in the best of spirits during the nine months of your pregnancy. These books also state that you need to limit the amount of fish you consume due to the possibility of mercury poisoning. Unfortunately, we cannot expect our waters to be entirely pure and the fear comes from the fact that no one can take that kind of a risk when one is pregnant. The other aspect that is worth mentioning is that most pregnancy books fail to mention that the seafood that is the best source of nutrients includes shellfish, fish eggs and fish organs. Cod liver oil is something that is to be avoided according to them since it can largely increase the level of vitamin A and D; more than what the pregnancy levels should be.

- *Organ Meats* — The pregnancy diet books available commonly will have you believe that the best options for vitamin A are green and red leafy vegetables. This is actually untrue. Fully formed physiologically-active vitamin A can only be obtained from animal sources. It is recommended that organ meats, like liver, should not be consumed. The fact, however, is that not only does the liver contain good levels of vitamin A, it is also a natural source of folic acid, a very important part of the development of fetal nervous system. Since organ meat is not one of the things that these books recommend, they tend to recommend consuming vegetables that are high in beta carotene. This is because beta carotene can be converted to vitamin A in the body. Well, they are right! Beta carotene can be converted into vitamin A in the body but what they fail to mention (unintentionally or intentionally) is that to make sure that the conversion does take place, there are various other factors that need to work out in the body. People who have digestive problems or problems of the thyroid may not be able to synthesize active vitamin from beta carotene easily. Lack of vitamin A also results in issues concerning absorption and assimilation of various nutrients that need vitamin A to be present.

- *Animal Fats* — If you go back in time or think about what your great grandmother said about fats, you may remember that her ideas about fats were completely different from what we think today. You can even speak to some older people in oriental societies who make sure that pregnant women in their families are pampered and fed large amounts of fat. In fact, most societies have special foods that are prepared especially for the pregnant women to ensure that her inner organs and skin are always lubricated and tight. While their specific reasons for feeding fat to pregnant women may not be fully understood, they were definitely doing the right thing. The fats play an important role in the physiology that takes place in the body. The sad part is that modern society has extended the fat-phobia that they have on to pregnant women too. And even at this stage when you should be eating a large amount of fat to ensure that your body stays healthy and that all the hormonal and chemical balances are maintained, we are told by the "so-called nutrition gurus" that too much fat is not good. By the way, it should be noted that fat consumption does not mean that you consume it to an extent where you exceed your required and optimum pregnancy weight. It is of extreme importance to stay within the limits of weight as recommended by your practitioner.

- *Egg Yolks* — Suggestions concerning egg are completely bizarre these days. They recommend that eggs should be limited to two per day at the maximum. Some suggest that the limit should be two to three per week and others recommend that the nutrient rich egg yolks should be thrown away and only the protein rich egg whites should be consumed. While some consider the egg yolks an issue due to its fat content, others feel that the added cholesterol is not good for health. All of this is not true. Eggs are a great source of protein and nutrients too, containing every vitamin except vitamin C.

- *Dairy Products* — While everyone will tell you that dairy products are the best source of calcium that you can have during pregnancy, what most of the modern books do not specify is that the pasteurized milk bought from regular stores cannot be absorbed easily by the stomach. In contrast it is recommended to stay away from raw milk because it may contain germs and viruses. Many people who may have an allergic reaction to milk will realize that this reaction occurs only when they consume pasteurized milk. Raw milk that is considered to be germ-filled by some is actually better in taste and deeper in color due to the high levels of vitamin A. Pasteurization reduces the level of vitamin C available to humans, converts the lactose in milk to beta-lactose and reduces the bio-availability of calcium too.

- *Carbohydrates* — Here again, while the basic recommendations regarding carbohydrate consumption is right, what is usually left out by most advisors is that whole grains should be used and that the nutritional value of the grains should be improved by soaking and sprouting. This method is used by many traditional communities and is the one I would suggest, if you incorporate whole grain into your diet. The soaking and sprouting method deactivates enzyme inhibitors and anti-nutrients like phytic acid and makes it healthier.

- *Protein* — Doctors will tell you that protein is required for the development of various tissues and muscles. Your placenta and the baby will benefit from your consumption of protein. It also helps in increasing the blood volume and prepares you for an easy lactation. Some of the sources of protein suggested include red meat, poultry, fish, cheese and milk, but in all of them, the lower fat version is recommended.

- *Vegetarian Diet* — A large number of books and literature available in book stores tells you that the vegetarian diet is great for you when you are pregnant. Don't fall for such talk just because the whole world seems to be going vegetarian these days. Most of the traditional are meat-consuming people and these people show far better internal and external health characteristics than the disease-laden modern people.

- *Supplements* — Supplements are considered to be a part of the pregnancy process. While some natural diets suggest that you should have fortified food and not take any calcium, it is interesting to note the ignorance of these authors who do not realize that fortified foods are nothing but supplemented foods. So taking regular food and popping in a calcium supplement is the same as using calcium fortified milk all the time.

There are some good aspects of modern books on pregnancy diets, like including evidence-based medicine, which makes it easier to figure out what information you should believe and what you should not. Otherwise one would wonder what kind of research they have done or what understanding they have of the human body to be recommending nutritional options that seem to go against the grain of everything that man (or shall we say woman) has been doing for years. Suggestions like the consumption of dark green leafy vegetables, whole grain, fresh fruits and vegetables and nuts are good and should be followed.

It almost seems like books that have been written about pregnancy diet have been compiled from various general books, on the fundamentals of nutrition, which are popular these days. With prevalence of obesity soaring high across the world, there is a lot of literature on how you need to reduce the consumption of fat, cholesterol and consume lean meat and processed and fortified beverages.

Even more ironic is the fact that the authors of the general nutrition books do not realize that the fundamentals they have based their recommendations on are completely wrong and that people are not likely to be able to achieve sustained levels of weight loss and good health simultaneously by following diets that deprive them of specific food groups.

The Weston A. Price Foundation recommends the following diet for women who are pregnant. This diet is based on the findings obtained from traditional communities that have a far higher proportion of normal birth than modern societies. In addition, this diet is extremely beneficial for overall health and immunity, too.

To start with, the diet expects that pregnant women who have scoliosis should avoid trans fatty acids, any kind of junk food or processed food, commercially fried food, refined sugar, refined grains, soft drinks, caffeine, alcohol, cigarettes and drugs (including those that may have been prescribed to you by overzealous physicians).

You should consume cod-liver oil for adequate levels of vitamin A and D, a quart of whole milk that is not pasteurized but obtained from pasture-fed cows, approximately 4 table-spoons of butter (in some form), 2 eggs (along with the egg yolk), coconut oil, lacto-fermented condiments, bone broths, soaked whole grain and loads of fresh fruits and vegetables. Fresh liver (about 3 to 4 ounces) should be consumed at least once or twice a week, fresh seafood (salmon, shellfish and fish eggs are particularly good) about two to four times a week and beef or lamb about two times a week (along with the natural fat).

In addition to this diet, you may also have some questions in mind concerning the specific kinds of things that you can eat or cannot eat. I have tried answering some of the questions that women have concerning diet and formulated do's and don'ts. I have also made sure that the questions are seen from a point of view that pertains to scoliosis and pregnancy. Understand that the diet that you need to consume is expected to be a natural one that is not tampered by the modern processes that are used in factories today. These diet recommendations for pregnancy and scoliosis ensure that you eat healthy to retain the health of your bones and skeleton along with the overall development of your child.

There is no doubt that I may not have been able to capture and address all the questions that you have. In case you have any doubts or suggestions, please feel free to write to me and we will try to address your particular issue.

- Many women want to know whether they should be taking prenatal medication because the amount of diet and natural vitamins that they consume in the first trimester are low due to morning sickness. While the logic does make sense, it is not recommended that you take any prenatal vitamin supplements because any such supplement contains chemicals and therefore may introduce the possibility of birth defects. The fact is that nature has a great way of managing these aspects. At the same time, you should make sure that you consume the right food in adequate quantities, even if you are feeling nauseous for some time and try to get in as much nutrition as you can for yourself and the baby.

- All sorts of soft drinks are banned when you are pregnant. In fact they do not form part of any healthy diet. Those who are used to drinking a beverage with their food may feel the need to substitute it with something else. Drinking kombucha or any kind of herbal tea or milk or fresh juice are great options that you can substitute for sodas. While herbal tea and milk are fine, do not drink kombucha if you have not had it before. This is because it can have side effects that you definitely do not want to see when you are pregnant.

- Fish is a great option for pregnant women and many women are extremely fond of sushi. However, it is best that you stay clear of sushi while you are pregnant and use other forms of lacto-fermented fish.

- One of the most nagging aspects of pregnancy is that you are not able to consume as much healthy food as you would want to during the first trimester when you are facing morning sickness. If you have been wondering how much food you are retaining inside and the amount that you are losing due to nausea and vomiting, you should try sipping raw milk through the day to keep the food down and ensure that you are able to eat. Warm the milk with some maple syrup or cinnamon and sip it regularly. Some other options that you have to fight nausea naturally include Swedish bitters or a little vinegar in water. If you are not able to keep food down, make bone broth, add in various vegetables and finely cut organ meat in small pieces to ensure that you get your daily dose of nutrition.

Before we get down to the specific aspects of each of the great nutrients that you should include in your pregnancy diet, consider some guidelines that apply to healthy eating. These guidelines will help you ensure that you are not only eating healthy for the baby but also for yourself. These guidelines will also help you in determining the specific points to pick up for yourself among all the recommendations that have been listed in the book. In effect, I have created guidelines that you can use to build up your own pregnancy diet based on specific principles and recommendations.

Without further ado, the guidelines that you need to follow during pregnancy are:

- Make sure that you evaluate your metabolic type and eat according to what you ancestors have been eating. For a change for these nine months try to think what your grandmother would have recommended and stick to that without trying your modern understanding of food.

- Buy a large amount of fresh whole food and consume them before they have a chance to get rot.

- Every bite that you eat counts. So eat fresh food that is nutrient rich. The more you can pack in a spoonful, the better it is. Avoid any kind of food that involves empty calories like refined white flour, sugar, starch, artificial colors and flavors.

- Do not stick to just a few fresh fruit or a few vegetables that you consume each day. Make it a point to consume a variety of options. You could boil the veggies, make them into a soup, steam them or sauté them if you like.

- Your main source of fluids should be water, fresh juices (not canned or those that you get in tetra packs or bottles) or milk. Processed fruit juices and sodas should be banned in the house for at least the time that you are pregnant and nursing.

- Make sure that you get in large amounts of traditionally fermented food to get a good quality of probiotics or good bacteria in your system. This will help you improve the absorption capabilities of your digestive system and you will be able to assimilate much more nutrients from the food that you are consuming.

- Do not forget to use meat broth made from bones of fish, chicken, beef or lamb. Use this in cooking to enhance the nutritional quality of the food.

- Eliminate the effect of phytic acid by sprouting whole grain before consuming it.

- The fats that you consume during these days should be healthy fats including extra virgin olive oil, butter, flax seed oil, coconut oil and other oils that are not refined chemically. Healthy fat can also be consumed in the form of animal fat from livestock that has been raised naturally.

We all know that as soon as you conceive, life begins. Right nutrition is required to grow this unique life and help it develop properly. Enough stress cannot be placed on the importance of nutrition during the early days of fetus in the womb. Even though people do not realize it, this is the stage that decides the fate of many people in the years to come as toddlers, children, teens and adults. It affects the brain, the kidneys, the cardiovascular system and the level of risk that you will be at concerning degenerative diseases.

The zygote (combination of the sperm and the egg) moves into the uterus to settle there in the first seven days of conception. Once this happens, it is called an embryo. Some people may be amazed at the fact that the heart of the embryo develops in 23 days and brainwaves can be recorded by the time the embryo is 40 days old. Within seven weeks the embryo is able to touch, frown, suck and hiccup too. After eight weeks, the embryo develops specific organs and is then called a fetus. At this time, a fetus has 4,000 out of the 4,500 body structures. At this stage, the fetus can suck his thumb, summersault and grip the umbilical cord.

Once the fetus moves into the third trimester, your child will be able to survive outside the womb too in case it is born prematurely. The baby grows by leaps and bounds in the last month especially the skeletal system. All this growth and development needs proper nutrients.

If you are wondering why we have moved into discussing fetal development of the child in the nutrition chapter, I need to explain that the embryo, fetus and the infant needs different levels of nutrition at different stages of development. The specific things that you need to eat, therefore, are also different. While you should be eating good nutrients throughout the nine months, you should place emphasis on some specific ones depending on the stage of pregnancy that you are in.

The Primitive Pregnancy Diet

Based on the study of primitive and traditional cultures, Weston A. Price Foundation has understood some basics concerning the diet that these groups followed. All communities that resided close to the sea ensured that their women consumed fish eggs. Milk was also consumed from grazing cows and it was actually encouraged that women should get pregnant at a time when the pastures were green and plenty. In some cultures men and women were expected to consume good milk for a few months before they get married.

Organ meat was another food that was a definite part of the pregnancy diet. This included moose thyroid, spider crabs and liver. Local plant food, fats and bone broth were consumed throughout the pregnancy.

While the primitive diet was not based on any research of specific ingredients that each of the foods contained, there was a lot of intelligence, knowledge and genius that went into it. Today you can find out that fish eggs are rich in vitamin B12, choline, selenium, calcium, magnesium, omega-3 fatty acids and cholesterol.

With the basic knowledge established, let us now have a look at specific nutrients and foods that are great for pregnant women with scoliosis.

Vitamin A

Vitamin A is required for the growing fetus so that the cells, tissues and organs can differentiate adequately. It also helps in the development of the communication system between the various organs and the brain because it creates the required network of nerves that are required for this communication. In addition to that, a lower level of vitamin A can also lead to a decrease in number of nephrons in the kidneys leading to weak kidneys at a later stage. Vitamin A is also required for the proper development of the ciliary hairs present in the lungs.

Vitamin A deficiency during pregnancy can cause a large number of specific conditions in fetus too. The offspring may have eye defects, displaced kidneys, harelip, cleft palate or abnormalities of the heart or the lungs. In laboratory animals, it has been shown to cause spontaneous abortion, eye defects of varying degrees, dental arches and lip distortions, displacement of ovaries, testis and kidneys, prolonged labor and even death of the mother.

The RDA of vitamin A that has been prescribed for a pregnant woman is 2600IU per day; only about 300 IU higher than that mentioned for a woman who is not pregnant. While the exact figures of the vitamin A included in the primitive pregnancy diet are unknown, it is expected that the nutrient would be consumed to the extent of 20,000 IU and higher. This assumption is based on the level of cod liver oil, milk, butter and eggs that are consumed as part of the pregnancy diet.

What is bizarre is that the modern day medical system warns pregnant women of consuming too much vitamin A because some claim that its excess may also lead to birth defects. The question that you probably need to ask yourself is why the pregnant women from traditional societies do not have children with large levels of birth defects if they consume such high levels of vitamins. The fact is that this observation about excess consumption of vitamin A through diet has been made on the basis of a single study, conducted by the scientists of the Institute of Medicine led by Dr. Kenneth Rothman of Boston, which was published in 1995. There were many things that were not right about the study. For example, the amount of vitamin A was calculated on the basis of the amount stored in the liver. This number was multiplied by two (since the liver is supposed to hold about half the vitamin A of the body) and they also divided the vitamin A absorption over the number of days of the last trimester (when the vitamin A is expected to be accumulated).

What the researchers at the Institute of Medicine assumed was that the amount of vitamin A found in the fetus may be used over a number of days for development. However, the nature of vitamin A is such that it is not meant to be stored, but used. The scientists also did not have a clue about the future health of the child in any manner possible. The study also observed over 23,000 women who were consuming more than 10,000 IU of vitamin A and observed that the offspring of these mothers were at a higher risk (4.8 times) of getting cranial-neural-crest defects. The large amount of vitamin A that was consumed by these women was also obtained from pills and supplements and not directly from food.

Contrary to the study mentioned above, there are a larger set of studies that have been done to prove that higher levels of vitamin A consumption is not harmful. These studies benchmark the birth defects among the incidence of birth defects in general. The incidence of birth defects was 3 to 4 percent and among those who consumed large levels of vitamin A these defects were about 3%; a figure that is at the lower end of the spectrum.

Vitamin E

In 1922, vitamin E was called "Fertility Factor X" because it was found that rats could not reproduce without it. Despite this fact, the scientists have been unable to ascertain completely why there is a definite need for vitamin E during pregnancy.

Simply because the scientists have not been able to prove it does not mean that we cannot see the reality as it exists. Vitamin E is important for human reproduction. Some great sources of vitamin E include nuts, seeds, fresh fruits and vegetables.

Vitamin D

When you reach the third trimester, you will start feeling a large amount of growth. This growth is visible from outside too and you should know that your baby is growing in terms of size with the skeleton becoming larger and stronger. In the last six weeks of pregnancy, about half the calcium that the child has at birth is infused into the skeleton of the child making vitamin D essential during this period. There is also some evidence that vitamin D helps in lung development and interacts with vitamin A for adequate growth. It has also been seen that the vitamin D levels in the blood of a newborn child is almost the same as their mothers.

Over the years, people have done numerous studies that have provided little clarity on the exact manner in which vitamin D works. This is because while one study explains the working of vitamin D in one way, the other one promptly negates the findings. In 1997, the Institute of Medicine stated that transfer of vitamin D from the mother to the fetus is minimal. They also stated that there is no need for a pregnant woman to take more vitamin D than that is required for women who are not pregnant. The conclusion seemed extremely illogical because the average amount of vitamin D recommended (200 IU per day) for women was low in the first place. What you may find even more appalling is that the American Academy of Pediatrics' Committee on Nutrition and its Section on Breastfeeding stated that the 400 IU of vitamin D that they recommended earlier was to be changed to 200 IU, the one that the Institute of Medicine had recommended.

Even more appalling is that newborn children were expected to be kept out of the sun and fully clothed while being taken into the sun. They also stated that breast milk is poor in vitamin D; not clarifying the situation. Contradictory guidelines, regarding the lower intake of vitamin D by the mothers and recommendations like keeping the baby out of the sun, are actually leading to further perplexity.

The Weston A. Price Foundation that has done a great empirical study of primitive cultures recommends 2000 IU per day of vitamin D. This can be obtained from cod liver oil, shellfish, butter and lard. Children in Finland who were supplemented with 2000 IU of vitamin D in the first year eradicated the risk of type 1 diabetes over the next

30 years. This study was done among 10,000 children.

Vitamin K

Not many scientists have a good understanding of the manner in which vitamin K works in the body or the manner in which it helps the growth of the fetus. Professionals hypothesize that the vitamin K dependent proteins like bone GLA protein and matrix GLA protein help in placing the calcium salts in the right place where they belong. This means that the calcium deposits in the bones and not in the area where soft tissue is expected to form. The enzymes that activate vitamin K dependent proteins are present in the fetus as early as the first trimester.

While we may not know what role vitamin K plays in the development of the fetus, we do know that severe issues can arise if there is a deficiency or blockage that does not allow the mother to use vitamin K. A mother who takes a drug called Warfarin during pregnancy will learn this the hard way. The drug that she might take to block the normal clotting mechanism may create a vitamin K deficiency. The baby born to such mothers have a stubbed nose at birth with development of cavities and plaques in the spine, leading to quadriplegia.

It is clear from this example that vitamin K is extremely necessary for proper proportions of the skeletal system and the nervous system as well. It is said that others who get vitamin K injections can transport the nutrient to the placenta; which then releases it to the fetus, based on the level that it is required. Some of the foods that have high levels of vitamin K include goose liver, natto and cheese. Butter and egg yolks also contain vitamin K to some extent.

DHA

DHA or docosahexaenoic acid is essential for the formation of neurons and brain lipids like phosphatidylserine. It is also a precursor to a compound that is synthesized to protect the neurons at a time when they are attacked by free radicals caused by stress. DHA can be created by the fetus, the infants and the adults from omega-3 fatty acid and alpha- linolenic acid that are found in plants oils. The rate of conversion is merely one percent in fetus and it stays at the same rate throughout life. A fetus gathers and stores DHA from the mother in its brain. This DHA can also be obtained from cod liver oil and fatty fish in large amounts.

Folate

The role of folate in pregnancy is probably the most familiar to most people. Folate is a type of vitamin B that is required for the proper production of DNA and we all know that new DNA is required to be produced for the child to grow. Folate also helps in preventing any nerve defects. It helps in increasing the weight of the child and prevents spontaneous abortion, mental retardation and deformations of the mouth.

The recommended levels of folate during pregnancy are considered to be 600 micrograms per day. Those who recommend this level also state that higher levels can result in dropping of the red blood cell count in the mother to low levels. It is also assumed that half the required amount comes from food and the remaining half needs to be supplemented.

The fact is that the amount of folate that is absorbed by the body depends highly on the level of zinc present. In addition to that, synthetic folate needs to be converted to usable folate. This conversion is normally limited to 200 micrograms per single dose. Over time, this capability may also drop to lower levels. Folate rich foods include liver, legumes and green leafy vegetables.

Choline

Low intake of choline is associated with a much higher (four times) risk of getting a neural tube defect. Choline is closely related to folate as it can get converted to a compound called betaine that works as a substitute for folate in some reactions.

In addition, you should also know that choline is directly involved in the development of the brain of the fetus. The development of cholinergic neurons that takes place from the 56th day of pregnancy until the end of three months requires choline. In fact, this is one element that you need to provide your child with, even after he is born and at least till he reaches the age of four. By this time, the production and differentiation of neurons and synapses are complete.

The studies done on rats that were fed high levels of choline showed that these rats produced offspring with 30 percent higher levels of visuo-spatial and auditory memory. The baby rats were observed until late in their life and it was seen that they did not develop any age-related senility and that they were far more resilient to the attack of neurotoxins.

While the RDA recommendation of choline for pregnant women is 425 milligrams per day, the above studies show that three times this amount can provide long lasting benefits to the offspring. Some of the foods that you can eat to augment your choline intake include liver, egg yolks, meats, nuts and legumes.

Glycine

An amino acid, glycine can be the limiting factor in the process of protein synthesis. The fetus can either draw glycine directly from the mother's blood or can use folate to make it from serine. It is important that the mother takes in adequate levels of glycine by consuming skin and bone broths.

Many people believe that the amount of focus that is laid on nutrition is not justified during pregnancy. Women who are afraid to put on weight and want to stick to their sickly weight loss diets even during pregnancy start believing the myth that the growth of their baby depends on their gene pool. Truthfully, they are right, but only to a small extent. The complete truth is that the genes limit the extent to which you can grow and develop in some specific areas. However, if the fetus is not nurtured with the right nutrients and minerals, it is likely that the child will have some sort of deficiency or deformation or retardation.

In a 1995 study, 62 cases of egg donors were studied. It was interesting to note that the birth-weight of a newborn did not correlate well with that of the egg donor, but was closely related to the weight of the recipient. The reasons are quite simple to understand. The environment in which the fetus is nurtured decides the level to which the child will flourish. If you consume less than 25 grams of protein and more than 265 grams of carbohydrate in the last part of the pregnancy, the weight of your newborn will be decreased. This kind of nutrition provided in the last trimester is also closely related to hypertension or high blood pressure at the age of 40 years and above.

Fatty Acids

Many researchers feel that the requirement for fatty acids is much higher in males. But not many people talk about over 300 Medline studies that have been done concerning the EFA (Essential Fatty Acids) requirement and status among women during the reproductive years. Studies have shown that the levels of essential fatty acids in women are critical for successful reproduction and lactation.

The EFA requirement for pregnant women is considered to be 6 percent of total calorific intake. Even a mild deficiency can hamper proper growth of the fetus. While some reports, like the FAO/WHO Rome Report, have recommended an increase in the consumption of total fat, especially in countries where malnutrition is a concern, the World Health Organization still reports a deficiency in fat intake in most developing countries.

Elongated EFA is a precursor to prostaglandins that are important for maintaining pregnancy. Researchers also report that there is a significant reduction in elongated EFA during pregnancy and coping with the high demand for the same, especially DHA is tough. Therefore, extra supplementation is a necessary aspect of a healthy pregnancy. The Dutch researcher, Dr. Gerard Hornstra has noted specifically that women should reduce their consumption of trans-fatty acids from 'industrial hydrogenation of edible oils'.

Some of the reliable sources of elongated omega-3 fatty acid include fatty fish like ocean salmon and tuna, cod liver oil and egg yolks. Organ meats from well fed hen and grass fed animals can also be used.

Vitamin B6

The role of vitamin B6 has been largely undermined in pregnancy to a large extent. Most of the times, women are asked to increase the intake of iron-rich food or they are given iron supplements to ensure that there is no risk of anemia during pregnancy. The fact is that the levels of iron and vitamin B6 fall drastically during the third trimester and there are great chances of concurrent vitamin B6 deficiency anemia. This can occur even when you have adequate supplies of iron in the blood.

Anemia during pregnancy can adversely affect the mental development of the fetus. The anemia caused by vitamin B6 cannot be differentiated from iron deficiency led anemia by blood tests and reports.

When the levels of vitamin B6 are lower in a pregnant mother, it is likely that the levels of vitamin B6 in breast milk will also remain low. The body does not have the ability to regulate the amount of vitamin B6 in breast milk in larger proportions. This means women who do not take adequate levels of vitamin B6 will not be able to produce breast milk that has the required levels. A group of researchers has concluded that a minimum of 3.5 to 4.9 mg of vitamin B6 is required to maintain adequate levels of vitamin B6 in mother's milk. This is double the amount that is considered to be the Recommended Daily Allowance.

Carbohydrates

Carbohydrates mainly consist of starches, sugars, cellulose and gums. Before you start understanding whether carbohydrates are a good thing to consume during your pregnancy or not, you need to know that there are two kinds of carbohydrates – simple and complex. Simple carbohydrates are those that are found in foods such as candy, fruits, baked foods and complex carbohydrates are the ones that you can find in vegetables, beans, whole grain and nuts. Simple carbohydrates are often considered an instant source of energy. The complex carbohydrates need more time to digest.

There is no doubt about the fact that carbohydrates provide energy for the body. It is also true that as they are digested along with the energy producing glucose, there is production of insulin, adrenaline and cortisol. These compounds can cause issues with diseases like diabetes, cancer, stroke, heart related complications, blood vessel issues, nerve disorders and more. We are also learning that these can have adverse effects on bone health.

Dr. Loren Cordain, a nutrition specialist believes that two to three servings of grain per day is the maximum serving that is required for an individual. You may have heard many vegetarian crusaders speak about how man was not supposed to eat meat and that we were originally meant to eat plants. But history shows us otherwise. The human system was not meant to consume foods high in carbohydrate but foods that are high in protein. This is something that can be ascertained by looking at some fossil studies that show that the stature of early farmers was much reduced. There was also a higher level of mortality in communities that were newly introduced to farming and agricultural based living.

In the words of Dr. Joseph Brasco, a medical doctor:

"In a review of 51 references examining human populations from around the earth and from differing chronologies, as they transitioned from hunter-gatherers to farmers, one investigator concluded that there was an overall decline in both the quality and quantity of life. There is now substantial empirical and clinical evidence to indicate that many of these deleterious changes are directly related to the predominately cereal-based diets of these early farmers. Since 99.99% of our genes were formed before the development of agriculture, from a biological perspective, we are still hunter-gatherers."

One has to merely look at the manner in which our diet has changed today to understand the amount of complications that women have in terms of pregnancy. The diet that the traditional and primitive man was used to was replete with proteins that were gained from sea food and meats. The fact however, was that these primitive women did all the housework on their own. They did not have nannies to take care of their children. They did not have dishwashers and washing machines and therefore kept themselves busy and exercised. They were not at a risk of becoming obese as we are today with all the gadgets that help us in completing the chores that we have.

Physical activity has reduced and the free time that we are able to get has been replaced with activities that do not demand much effort. Sitting on the computer and networking or completing our jobs does not create as much exercise as cleaning the house and managing children does.

With lack of exercise and an additional amount of carbohydrates that we eat due to processed foods and refined grains, the result is larger amounts of insulin secretion. While insulin helps with sugar metabolism, it also stimulates fat accumulation around the waist. It stimulates the appetite and increases the chances of heart diseases, scoliosis and cancer. Insulin is also known to increase the production of C-reactive protein that speeds up inflammation and aging. High levels of insulin in the blood may also lead to an inability to store calcium and magnesium, causing a large amount of damage to the bones.

The amount of sugar that we consume these days causes many issues for everyone, especially for pregnant women. While there is nothing wrong with sugar per se, the kind of carbohydrate-rich foods that we consume are stripped of all the protein, vitamins and minerals. Digesting refined sugars without the presence of other nutrients is impossible. Incomplete metabolism of carbohydrates causes production of pyruvic acid. This starts accumulating in the brain, the central nervous system and the red blood cells. These poisonous metabolites interfere with cell respiration, causing them to die.

Over-indulgence in carbohydrates is the real cause of the obesity that we are seeing around the world. Everyone seems to blame the fat content of their food for this phenomenon. If you could cut out sugars from your diet and ensure that you consume whole grain (instead of refined ones), you could ensure that you stay healthy, fit and free of toxins too.

It is also extremely important that you understand what is good for your body and what is not. Many people get confused with labels that state "no sugar" and assume them to be a healthier option. Beware of such things, especially when you are pregnant because these foods, on the supermarket shelf, can contain additives and derivatives that you cannot afford to consume. Some of these foods contain aspartame, a sugar substitute that is known to be cancerous. Other foods that are labeled with corn syrup, corn oil, corn meal, corn-starch, xanthan gum and maltodextrin are also more or less equally dangerous for you and your baby. Corn sweeteners are being used rampantly in the western world as substitutes for sugar, but it has been adequately maligned. Today, it is one of the most common reasons for obesity and diabetes.

Excess carbohydrates produce higher levels of insulin that in turn lead the body to produce excess cortisol that is responsible for demineralization of bones, among other things. When the bone minerals are washed away along with the connective tissues, it leads to osteoporosis and degenerative disc disease. Considering your scoliosis and the stage of life you are in, bone health is extremely important and you should ensure that you are in good health in order to be able to carry the weight of your child for the complete nine months with the least agony.

The added information that you need to have when deciding on the pregnancy diet that you shall follow, is that supplementing the calcium and magnesium requirement of your body by drinking milk and consuming yogurt and dairy products does not help to a large extent. This is because the additional intake of carbohydrates continuously depletes the body of minerals like calcium, magnesium, manganese, chromium, zinc, cobalt and copper. This is mainly because the process of digesting sugars causes acidity in the system leading to a depletion of these essential minerals.

But this does not mean that your body does not need carbohydrates. The best carbs to consume are the ones present in vegetables. Vegetables provide a good source of the carbohydrates that we need. Since the vegetables that you eat have a fair amount of fiber in them, they ensure that the digestion is slower. While this explanation is true for carrots and corn, it does not really apply to potatoes, especially if they are deep fried (as in the case of French fries). Potatoes are exceptionally high in carbohydrates and they do not contain the adequate level of fiber to ensure slow digestion.

The best option available in vegetables is organically grown vegetables. Do make sure that you buy organic product that is fresh. If this is something that you cannot procure in your area, then you should opt for fresh fruits and vegetables. Canned and frozen vegetables are not really a healthy choice.

Another myth that you need to be aware of is that all fruits are healthy. There is no doubt that fruits are a good source of fiber and some of the minerals that you may need during pregnancy. Do remember that they do contain fructose in high quantities and fructose is a sugar. The body therefore responds to fructose just like it does to sugar. So while you should consume fruits during your pregnancy, you need to limit the consumption to ensure that you do not consume large quantities.

Protein

Everyone knows that protein is important for the growth and repair of the body. This is the reason why they are called the 'building blocks' for nutrition, growth and repair. Proteins are actually amino acids that link together in varying combinations to form enzymes that can be used for different functions.

While vegetables do contain some amino acids, only animal products can provide all the eight essential amino acids. Legumes are high in vegetable protein and also provide fiber and minerals. They do not contain all the essential amino acids that the body requires. Therefore, animal protein is a necessity if you want to ensure that you get complete protein nutrition.

Many people may warn you about the dangers of eating too much beef or red meat. The problem does not lie with the meat, but the manner in which this meat is processed and brought to you. Until the middle of the 20th century, the cows that were later slaughtered for beef consumption were fed on grass. These cows were fed for a period of four to five years. These days the cows are fed on corn or grain and they are readied for the market in 14 to 16 months. This is great for business but definitely not great for the people who consume this kind of meat.

Cows fed on grains and corn, are more likely to get some kind of disease. Cows are ruminants and their systems are not created in a manner that can allow grain digestion. The stomach has the right juices to ferment grass but not grain. Cows raised on grass are also leaner. Grass fed beef also provides you with the extra omega-3 fatty acids that you need when you are pregnant.

The protein that you should consume when you are pregnant should come from sea food and grass fed cow beef. The latter has proven to be a good source of omega-3 fatty acid, conjugated linoleic acid, beta carotene, higher levels of vitamin A and vitamin E, along with no risk of bovine infections.

There is also no doubt that fish and seafood are the best options for a pregnant mother to get all her protein. The problem here again is not with the fish per se but the manner in which it is reared and grown. Most of the fish you see in the supermarket is likely to be factory farmed. Since these fish farmers are mainly concerned with their profits large amounts of fish are kept in small confined areas. The overcrowding can cause disease and injuries to the fish. To ensure that they do not develop infections, the fish are fed with antibiotics and chemicals. Some are even given hormones and drugs and yet others are genetically modified. There are also various other tricks that these fish farmers use to make the fish pinker in order to sell them more easily and at a higher price. For example, farmed salmon is often given canthaxanthin and astaxanthin to make their flesh look pinker. Natural salmon that lives in the sea, feed on shrimp and krill, something that makes their flesh pink naturally without the need for chemicals. The safest fish to eat if you do not have access to natural fish include Wild Pacific Salmon, Snapper, Striped Bass, Sardines, Haddock and Pacific Flounder.

Another source of great protein is eggs. If you have been told to steer clear of eggs because they are full of cholesterol or they cause heart diseases then maybe you need to stop listening to these people. Eggs are a great source of all kinds of minerals that you need except for vitamin C. They have large amounts of vitamin A and vitamin D that fight against free radicals. They are also high in protein; the building block, required in large amounts by the mother, for her fetus.

You need to be careful about the eggs that are produced artificially. You should ensure that the eggs that you eat when you are pregnant are from hens that are fed on their natural food. Eggs should either be boiled or consumed as 'sunny side up' since this ensures that the yolk does not come in contact with the white, something that oxidizes it.

Fats

The most important things that we need to discuss are the myths associated with fats. This is also because there are many myths that are associated with this element of the food pyramid. So here are some of the things that you may have heard about very often, making you believe them automatically.

- *Fat consumption causes heart disease* — Animal fats in particular are blamed for the level of cholesterol and saturated fats that they have. The incidence of heart diseases in America increased drastically between the period of 1920 and 1960. This was the time when consumption of animal fat declined and that of hydrogenated and industrially processed vegetable fats increased (USDA-HNIS).

- *Arteries get clogged with saturated fats* — There are studies that prove that the fats that clog arteries are unsaturated. This proportion is as high as 74 percent and therefore defies everything that is said about saturated fat clogging arteries.

- *Animal fat can cause cancer* — You only have to look at the decreasing amounts of animal fat consumption in the country to know that this is not the truth. People are consuming lesser levels of animal fat with relatively large proportion becoming vegetarians and vegans. Yet the incidence of cancer has not reduced, but only skyrocketed.

- *Low fat diets can help you feel better* — This is a myth that people confuse with exercise. While getting on an exercise routine will help you feel better about yourself, consuming lower levels of fat have been associated with depression, fatigue, irritability, feelings of suicide and psychological problems.

- *The cave-man diet was low in fat* — This cannot be further from the truth. Primitive people did not consume hydrogenated fats but a large amount of animal fat from fish, shellfish, sea mammals, land birds, pigs, sheep, goats and nuts. (Abrams, Food & Evolution 1987).

This said there are some kinds of fat that are not healthy. These are the fats that can actually cause the diseases and conditions that are otherwise associated with fats in general. Some of the areas of concern include cancer, heart disease, compromised immune system, sterility, learning disabilities, growth problems and osteoporosis.

Partially hydrogenated oils and hydrogenated oils are not good for health. In addition to these, industrially processed liquid oils like soy oil, corn oil, safflower oil, cottonseed oil and canola also are not healthy. Even fats and oils that are heated to high temperatures while frying are not good for re-use.

Hydrogenation solidifies liquid oils and helps in increasing the shelf life of the fat. It also adds flavor to the food. Some of the common foods in which hydrogenated oils are added include margarine, crackers, bakery items, biscuits, snack foods and processed foods.

Ask anyone and you are likely to be told that saturated fats should be blamed for all the health-related problems that one is facing. But the reality is completely different. Vegetable oils that are processed are the real cause of all the problems since they include high levels of free radicals that cause all the diseases.

Saturated fats are good for human beings because we are warm blooded animals. We do not function at room temperature. These fats provide the stiffness that is required for our cell membranes and tissues to remain healthy. Saturated fats also increase immunity and help in better inter-cell communication. They help the lungs function better and ensure that the kidneys and hormonal system works properly.

Another very important aspect that a pregnant mom should know is that fats are extremely helpful in the working of the nervous system. Therefore, to ensure a good nervous system for your baby, you need to consume the right amount of saturated fat.

While fats may be portrayed as demons in western society, one only has to look at the Inuit diet to know differently. More than 50 percent of the daily calorific intake in an Inuit diet comes from fat and yet their levels of heart diseases are no different (and indeed lower) than Americans or Canadians. At the same time, what is important is that the fat that these people consume comes from wild animals and not farm fed animals that are grown and fed on chemical laden food or drugs.

A great source of good saturated fat is coconut. Among the three different types of saturated fats, coconut contains the healthiest type of saturated fat. A study conducted in 2004 and published in Clinical Biochemistry showed that coconut oil lowers total cholesterol and LDL (the bad cholesterol).

The medium chain fatty acids (MCFA) that are abundant in coconut oil can be digested easily. It goes directly to the liver, where it is converted to energy instead of being stored as fat. This method puts less work-load on the pancreas and the digestive system for digestion.

A large part of the research that was conducted by Dr. Price of the Weston A. Price foundation refers to the "fat-soluble activators". These are vitamins, namely vitamin A, vitamin D and vitamin K which are catalysts for mineral absorption. This means that a large part of what we eat cannot be absorbed properly if we do not have these "activators" in the required quantity. Traditional diets contained more than 10 times the amount of these nutrients.

The great thing is that modern research also validates the findings of Dr. Price. We know that vitamin A is necessary for mineral and protein metabolism and in the prevention of birth defects. It is also necessary for proper development of the fetus and infants, in addition to the production of stress and sex hormones, thyroid function and healthy eyes and bones.

Vitamin D is essential for healthy bones, muscle tone, proper functioning of the nervous system, reproductive health and various psychological issues. Vitamin K, on the other hand, helps with proper skeletal development, reproduction and protection against calcification and inflammation of arteries. There is also a belief that these vitamins work in a synergistic manner.

When you eat saturated fat along with these vitamins, you ensure that there is optimal physical and mental development of your child. Vitamin A can be found in animal sources like beef, fatty fish, cod liver oil, egg yolk and dairy products. A precursor of vitamin A is beta carotene that can be found in green leafy vegetables and brightly colored vegetables like carrots. Vitamin D is produced by the body when it is exposed to the sun. Vitamin K is also made by your body with the use of beneficial bacteria in the intestines. This is why consuming fermented foods like natto and kefir are beneficial. Other foods that contain vitamin K include cabbage, cauliflower, spinach and broccoli.

Probiotics

Probiotics are extremely essential if you want to remain disease-free during the months of your pregnancy. This is because about 80 percent of the immune system resides in the gastrointestinal tract. There are more than 500 species of bacteria that live in this tract at any given point in time. There are about a 100 trillion bacteria living inside you. This is more than 10 times the total number of cells that you have in your entire body.

The ideal balance between good and bad bacteria is 85% to 15%. Probiotics help in increasing the number of good bacteria, thereby balancing the flora in your body. People have used fermented foods like yogurt to increase the level of good bacteria in their body. In India, people still consume a yogurt based drink called lassi before every meal. Bulgarians also consume a large amount of fermented milk and kefir and they are known for their longevity. In Asian cultures, fermentation of turnip, cabbage, eggplant, cucumbers, squash, onions and carrots is still common.

Along with probiotics, Kefir contains Tryptophan, an amino acid that can have a relaxing effect on the central nervous system. It also contains large amounts of calcium and magnesium and is a rich source of vitamin B12, B1 and vitamin K. Fermented food or cultured food are foods that are partially digested by enzymes, fungi or good bacteria. This makes the nutrients in the food more bio-available than otherwise. Making cultured food such as saurkraut is easy. You can shred cabbage and other vegetables and pack them into an airtight container. Leave it for fermenting in warm temperature for a few days. During the fermentation stage the sugars will get reduced to starches and lactic acid. Once the fermentation has been done, you can reduce the level of fermentation by putting these vegetables in a refrigerator. Over time the vegetables become 'pickled' in a manner of speaking. The enzymes in the fermented foods also help digest the food that is eaten along with them too.

Making Your Own Kefir

Kefir, which literally translated means "feel good" in Turkish, is an ancient cultured, enzyme-rich food filled with friendly micro-organisms that help balance your "inner ecosystem" to maintain optimal health and strengthen immunity.

Ingredients

- 50 grams (1¾ oz) of kefir grains or kefir starter culture
- 500 ml (1 pint) fresh milk

Preparation:

- Remove kefir grains from previous batch of starter, using a sieve or colander.
- Shake kefir grains to remove excess kefir. Rinsing is not necessary (but optionally, rinse in fresh milk).
- Place kefir grains in glass jar or jug with fresh milk. Generally, keep a ratio of kefir grains to milk of about 1:10.
- Set aside to ferment at room temperature for up to 24 hours.

Note: Non-milk kefir can be made from sugary water, fruit juice, coconut juice, rice milk, or soy milk. However, the kefir grains will stop growing in these liquids, so it is best to only use excess kefir grains or powdered kefir starter for this.

Two Cultured Vegetables Recipes

Traditional Sauerkraut

Ingredients:

- One fresh medium-sized cabbage, red or green
- Non-chlorinated water
- Vegetable "starter culture"

Preparation:

- Shred the cabbage either by hand or with a food processor.
- Place the shredded cabbage in a large bowl.
- Pound the cabbage.
- Mix 1 packet of vegetable culture starter to the filtered water.
- Place pounded cabbage and juices in a medium sized glass jar. Press down firmly on the cabbage while pouring cultured water to the jar until cabbage is fully submerged. The mixture should be at least one inch from the top of the jar.
- Cover the jar and let it sit for 3 to 7 days at room temperature.
- After it is fermented, store it in the refrigerator.

Once in the fridge, it can last 2-3 months due to the preservation method used. Vegetables such as carrots, cauliflower, wakami, chili and ginger can be added to make it more interesting.

Kimchi (Korean Sauerkraut)

Ingredients:

- 1 head of cabbage, cored and shredded
- 1 bunch of green onions, chopped

- 1 cup of carrots, grated
- 1/2 cup of daikon radish, grated (optional)
- 1 tablespoon ginger, freshly grated
- 3 cloves of garlic, peeled, crushed and minced
- 1/2 teaspoon of dried chili flakes
- 1 tablespoon of ocean sea salt, i.e. "Celtic Sea Salt or Himalayan"
- 1 packet of vegetable culture starter

Preparation:

- Place vegetables, ginger, red chili flakes, ocean sea salt and water made with the starter culture in a bowl and pound it with a wooden mallet to release the juices.
- Put it all in wide-mouth jar with a tight-fitting lid.
- Press down firmly with a mallet until the juices rise to the top of the mixture. The juice should completely cover the vegetables, and the top of the juices and mixture should be at least 1 inch below the top of the jar, to allow room for expansion.
- Screw the cover on tightly and keep it at room temperature (68 to 77 degrees Fahrenheit) for 3 days (72 hours).
- After 3 days, it should be kept in the refrigerator or some other cold place.

Omega 3

One nutrient that has been neglected a lot in modern diets is omega-3 fatty acid. Omega-3 fatty acids are not only important for conception, but these are also important for the maintenance of pregnancy. While traditional diets contained fatty acids so that the proportion of omega-6 to omega-3 was 1:1, modern day diets have far too much omega-6. The ratio falls somewhere between 50:1 and 20:1. What we, therefore, need to do is increase the amount of omega-3 and reduce omega-6. Some fatty acids that are high in omega-3 include Alpha Linolenic Acid (ALA), Eicosapentaenoic acid (EPA) and Docosahexaenoic acid (DHA).

ALA can be obtained from plant sources like flax seeds and walnuts but EPA and DHA can be obtained mainly from marine life. You can also improve the ration of omega-6 to omega-3 by changing the kind of meat you consume. Grass fed cattle tends to have an omega-6 to omega-3 ratio of 0.16:1; considered ideal for a healthy diet. Not only does this ratio help in fighting degenerative bone health issues, but it also helps in maintaining the normal heart function, reducing inflammation and providing proper nervous development of the fetus.

At the cost of being repetitive, but for the sake of summarizing, below are some points that you need to keep in mind to be able to create the best pregnancy diet for yourself.

- Do not put faith in what the modern pregnancy books tell you, without thinking for yourself. Many of these books are based on myths that have been brought to us over the ages. In addition, they are also influenced by what the manufacturers of various food products would like us to believe.

- Go back to the primitive diet that our ancestors used and you will be thankful one day that you went back to your roots.

- Do not assume that all kinds of fats are bad and unhealthy. Make sure to have adequate levels of saturated fat so that the "activators" can do their job well.

- Fatty acids in the right proportion are extremely important.

- The best way to ensure a good diet is to "go back to the basics" and eat meat that comes from naturally-raised animals such as grass-fed animals and wild-caught fish that is not grown in farms.

CHAPTER 12

EXERCISES TO FOLLOW DURING PREGNANCY

A woman's body goes through a lot of changes when she delivers a baby. While some accept the changes that happen in our bodies while they are pregnant, there are many of us who are not able to accept or live through the time that it takes for the body to come back in shape after delivery. Sometimes it seems that the media is to be blamed for all the unrealistic images of expectant mothers coming back into shape as soon as the baby is delivered. But if you are well-read, then you might already know that this is not to be believed.

There are various benefits of exercising during pregnancy and after delivery. Physically, you shall be able to achieve better lumbo-pelvic stability, have a proper stance and have stronger muscles to get them back to their original sizes. You shall also be able to take care of the back, abdominal and pelvic area; an aspect that you need to be particularly careful about due to your scoliosis. Exercise has also been known to help with better immunity, better sleep quality (and you need to improve on quality since the quantity of sleep will reduce as you get into your third trimester and will reduce even further after you deliver), better digestion and quicker healing.

But before you delve onto the specific exercises that you must perform during pregnancy and post-pregnancy, it is important to understand what really happens to the structure of the body especially in relation to our posture, hip bone (pelvis) and spine.

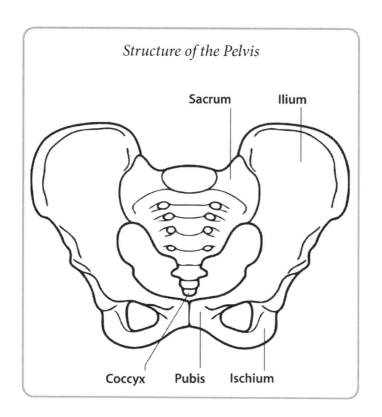

Structure of the Pelvis

Sacrum   Ilium

Coccyx   Pubis   Ischium

The pelvis comprises of five bones – the ilium or the wing shaped part of the pelvis, the ischium or the thick lower part of the pelvis that leads to the part called 'sitting bones', the pubis or the front of the pelvic region where the two bones meet, the sacrum or the triangular-shaped bone that is made of 5 fused vertebrae and the coccyx that is made from 4 fused vertebrae.

The pelvis mainly has two important joints:

- *Symphysis pubis (SP)* — This is situated at the front of the pelvis, where the 2 pubic bones meet. It is separated by a cartilage that is generally 4mm wide. This joint does not provide any movement, except during pregnancy.

- *Sacroiliac joints (SIJ)* — These are the joints that attach the spine to the pelvis. Since they support the weight of the upper body and also bears the impact that the lower body transmits while walking or running, these joints are considered to be the strongest joints in the body,. These joints are considered to be synovial joints since the fluid allows gliding movement. However, by the age of 30, these joints start to turn into cartilaginous joints.

Since these joints are not supposed to move too much, there are a couple of closure mechanisms to ensure that the joints stay in place. These are called form closure and force closure. Form closure is associated with the structure of the ligaments, bones and joints and force closure with the activation or movement of muscles and fascia. The triangular sacrum located in between the two hip bones provides form closure and pelvic muscles provide force closure, helping in compression of the joints to provide some mobility.

When you are pregnant, the level of laxity in the joints increases. The pelvic outlet starts to enlarge in size to allow for delivery. One of the major issues that one in every five pregnant women face is pelvic girdle pain. This is a term used to refer to any kind of lower back pain or pelvic issues. Since they can cause significant distress during pregnancy and disability too, these symptoms need to be taken seriously.

Relaxin is the hormone responsible for making the pelvic bones more mobile than they generally are. This is a hormone that is produced in pregnant and non-pregnant women. In non-pregnant woman or those who are in their first trimester, the Relaxin is produced by the corpus luteum (a yellow mass that is left behind in the ovary after ovulation). However, as soon as you enter your second trimester, the production of Relaxin is taken over by the placenta and the decidua. The placenta stops producing Relaxin after it is delivered.

Since Relaxin provides a higher level of movement in the pelvic area and also the lower back area, it is necessary that the exercises that are done during pregnancy be done with a lot of care. I have detailed some points that you need to keep in mind at all times. These are the aspects that need to be remembered when you are exercising during pregnancy or post-delivery. This is because people tend to ignore the lingering effects of Relaxin that can continue to cause issues in the lower back and pelvic area.

- All exercises should be performed within the normal range of motion.

- It is also necessary that speed be given extra thought since long levered fast movements can lead to over-stretching. Therefore activities such as kick boxing, Tae-Bo, karate and other forms of exercises that involve quick movements should be avoided.

- Even while doing yoga exercises that do not involve jerky or quick movements, the range of movement should be kept in mind. Over-stretching is extremely likely if care is not taken.

- The body alignment while doing specific exercises should be kept in mind. Locking knees or elbows in any exercise or any posture is not recommended.

- A tall upright stance should be maintained at all times.

- The spine should always be in the neutral position.

- When performing repetitive cardio exercises, like the cross trainer or the stepper, it is important that you keep an eye on the time.

- Cycling is something that you should avoid during pregnancy and even after delivery since it can cause discomfort in the symphysis pubis and sacro-iliac joints.

- Excessive stretching needs to be avoided. This is something that you may want to do in post-partum period, but you need to wait for at least 16 to 20 weeks after delivery. Trying to go beyond normal joint range can affect joint stability and the over-stretching can sometimes lead to permanent laxity.

- All high impact activities need to be put on hold till about a month after delivery. This increased pressure on the joints can put a lot of stress on the knees, ankles, pelvis and also the spine. Running should be avoided completely till about a month after delivery and best avoided if you have a severe curve.

- If you have been training consistently and maintaining your exercise level during pregnancy, it can be continued at about 70 percent of the pre-pregnancy load. Aspects that need to be avoided include over-use of an unstable or lax joint, working on a base that is not stable or starting your work-outs with heavy weights.

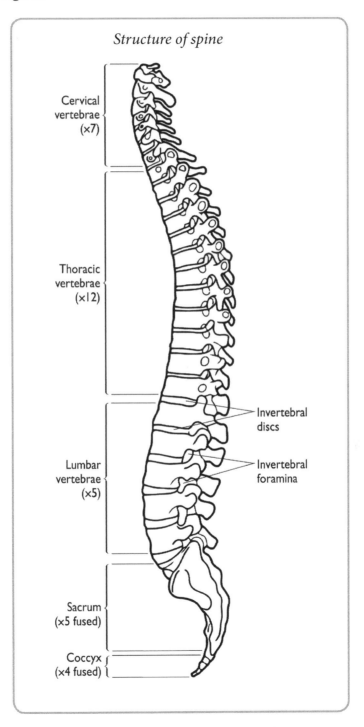

Structure of spine

Cervical vertebrae (×7)

Thoracic vertebrae (×12)

Lumbar vertebrae (×5)

Intervertebral discs

Intervertebral foramina

Sacrum (×5 fused)

Coccyx (×4 fused)

The pressure that pregnancy puts on the spine is too large. This is why special care needs to be taken in order to protect the spine from harm in any way. The spine is made up on 33 bones; 24 of which are separate, 5 of which fuse to form the sacrum and the remaining 4 merge to make the coccyx. The small sections of the spine are separated by intervertebral discs that are made of fibrocartilage. This cartilage provides a cushion to the movements of the spine that are so regular and excessive in nature. They also provide the cushion and shock absorption capabilities that are required to protect the spinal cord from any kind of shock.

Postrual Changes During Pregnancy

The forward pull of the abdomen may displace the pelvis forward. To compensate for the forward shift and maintain balance, the upper body sways backwards, creating a high lumbar lordosis.

Alternately, the loss of tone in the rectus abdominis reduces the ability to maintain correct pelvic alignment and result in an anterior tilt.

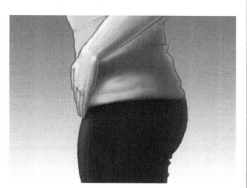

Neutral Pelvis

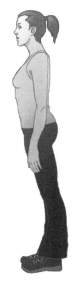

Correct posture

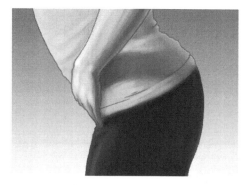

Anterior Pelvic Tilt

It is important to maintain the correct spinal posture at all times and especially during pregnancy. This is called the neutral position. When the cervical and lumbar parts of the spine are curved inwards and the thoracic part is curved outwards, the pressure on the spine is equally distributed causing the least amount of stress. In this position most of the support is provided by the bones of the spine and minimal muscle support is required.

Correct position of the spine can help in better neuromuscular efficiency, elimination of pain, prevention of injury, better circulation, better flexibility, efficient breathing and release of tension.

It is normal for the spinal alignment to change when you are pregnant. There is a higher level of flexibility and elasticity in the ligaments of the spine and the large abdomen creates a forward pull which leads to an anterior pelvic tilt. These changes in the body make it difficult to maintain the neutral spinal position. The added weight of the growing breasts also makes it tough to maintain a proper stance.

Musculoskeletal Pregnancy Changes

No specific normal posture has been defined for pregnant women. What really happens when you are pregnant is that some of the posture imbalances get exaggerated. Sometimes the pull that you feel due to a growing abdomen can lead to the pelvis moving forward. This is compensated by moving the upper body backwards; something that creates lumbar lordosis.

There is also a loss of tone in the rectus abdominus. Therefore, the ability to maintain a correct pelvic stance is also reduced leading to an anterior tilt. If the baby is on one side, there is a chance of lateral flexion. In the third trimester the lower rib-cage flares and the uterus rises to the upper abdomen. This reduces thoracic mobility.

All these changes have an impact on the kind of exercises that you should do during pregnancy.

Abdominal Muscles and the Changes in them During Pregnancy

The spine and the pelvic bones are not the only parts that are affected during pregnancy. The whole body goes through significant changes that include significant changes in the bones, muscles and various systems of the body.

The abdominal muscles help in supporting various parts of the spine including the pelvic and the lumbar regions. It also supports the organs in these areas. The abdominal muscles are also responsible for flexing and curling the trunk and maintaining correct pelvic alignment. They help in expulsive movements like vomiting and excretion, not to forget their role in pushing the baby out during delivery.

During pregnancy, the abdominal muscles undergo a lot of stretching in order to accommodate the growing baby. Relaxin plays a role in this stretching too. There is also a separation of the recti muscles, a normal phenomenon that takes place in the third trimester in about 66 percent of the women.

Some women believe that the damage to abdominal muscles during a caesarean section is excessive and almost impossible to repair. This is however not true, since the muscles are not cut during the procedure.

Recovery of the abdominal muscles starts to occur a few days after the delivery. The wide separation of the muscles also starts to reduce. By 8 weeks, the reduction in the gap is at its peak and this is where a plateau is reached in most cases. After this stage, exercises are required to reduce the gap further. Exercises to strengthen abdominal muscles can start almost immediately after delivery. In fact women should start doing these exercises within 24 hours of the delivery itself. Pelvic tilting and Level 1 Transversus Abdominis exercises are something that most hospitals educate about before discharging the mother.

Structure of the Pelvic Floor

The pelvic floor is made up of muscles and fascia. It is formed out of various layers – the deepest fascia layer, the muscular levator ani layer, the perineal membrane that connects the urethra and the vagina to the pelvic walls and the superficial perineal muscles that are arranged in the form of the figure eight.

The pelvic floor muscles support the pelvic organs and help in urinary and fecal continence. They help in controlling the sudden urge to void and help in turning the baby into right position required for a comfortable delivery. During pregnancy, the pelvic floor muscles change due to the increased weight that they need to support.

The first vaginal delivery can cause a fair amount of muscle and nerve damage. The muscles of the pelvic floor need to stretch completely in order to allow for the baby to descend. Often the perineum undergoes trauma due to tearing or episiotomy.

Pregnancy and Structure of the Breasts

We all know that the breasts go through a large number of changes during pregnancy. This is a change that you will start to see in the first trimester itself. Breast tissue growth is stimulated by higher levels of estrogen, progesterone and relaxin.

The breasts begin to enlarge and get filled with milk as there is abundance of milk. As the baby begins to suck, the engorgement reduces but it also triggers more production of prolactin. As the prolactin levels increase, the estrogen levels reduce; something that leads to absence of the menstrual cycle. This causes the ovarian functions to be suppressed causing some menopausal symptoms like hot flushes, night sweats and reduced vaginal secretions.

Breastfeeding also leads to a significant impact on the bone mineral content of the body. The body loses about 5 percent bone minerals in the first 3 months. This is because estrogen maintains the correct balance of bone formation and resorption, helping in calcium absorption and reducing loss of calcium through the kidneys. In the event of no estrogen production, these functions are compromised leading to weaker bones during this time.

This is why it is essential that breastfeeding women continue to supplement their intake of calcium in as many ways as possible. The loss of bone density carries on for about 6 months after which it stops. At the same time, it has been seen that the bone density takes about 6 months more to recover after you stop breastfeeding your baby.

The specific posture that one adopts during breastfeeding also impacts the amount of stress that the spine has to tolerate. This can cause a chronic ache in the neck and shoulders. Many women feel that exercising during the breastfeeding period is not a good idea. On the contrary, weight bearing and resistance training can increase muscle mass so that various other structures can be supported. Aerobics and resistance exercises can also slow down bone density loss.

Breastfeeding is an activity that utilizes about 500 calories per day on an average. The manner in which fat is utilized for this purpose also helps in weight loss. However, drastic dieting or intense exercises may cause the quality of the milk to deteriorate.

You must keep some things, concerning exercises, in mind when you are breastfeeding.

- Make sure that you express milk or feed before exercising. Not only will this reduce the load in the breasts but it will also prevent leakages. Large and full breasts are likely to feel uncomfortable.

- Make sure that the bra that you wear has adequate support. This will also help in preventing overstretching. Do not continue to wear the nursing bra that you use on a regular basis. Change into your sports bra to reduce the bounce and to obtain better shock absorption value.

- Reduce the range of movement that is required for arm exercises. Do not compromise on body position and joint alignment to try to lift higher levels of weight. On the other hand, make sure that you start with light weights.

- Roll a towel under the breasts when doing exercises that are required in the prone position.

Exercising During Pregnancy

Exercising during pregnancy is important for every pregnant woman. If you do not exercise, you are likely to become increasingly less fit as the months go by. As you become heavier, initiating exercise will also become tougher. Therefore, it is a good idea to start exercising right from the beginning.

Exercise can help you combat the lack of fitness that you are likely to feel as the months go by. It will help you feel more energetic, help you sleep better and will also ensure that your mood swings are managed better. Exercise also helps you strengthen muscles so that you can manage the imbalances caused by the growing belly, reduce the backaches that you get and helps you get back into pre-pregnancy shape faster.

Irrespective of how good you feel, you should make sure that you visit your practitioner and have a word with him about the exercises that you plan to do.

Pregnant women with scoliosis have a higher need to exercise since they can benefit a lot from the spine support that exercise provides. The increased weight starts to put a larger amount of pressure on the spine and exercise can help reduce the amount of stress that the spine has to endure. In addition to that, the additional ligament laxity that the hormonal changes cause can add to the backache and pain.

Pregnant women can do aerobics, calisthenics and water workouts too. Aerobics are rhythmic repetitive movements that are strenuous enough to require higher levels of oxygen. Some of the aerobic exercises that you can do are brisk walking, jogging, bicycling and swimming. Calisthenics are light gymnastic movements that tone muscles. These can help in gaining better support and improving posture. Some of these exercises have been developed especially for pregnant women and these can help provide relief from backaches too. Make sure that you do not practice calisthenics that have been developed for the general public. You must have heard about water workouts for pregnant women and there are various classes that you can join for the same. These are less stressful on the joints due to the lift that the water provides you. You can also take on yoga exercises that are specially meant for pregnant women. These can be extremely good for building endurance and improving posture.

It is important that you choose the right exercises for yourself during pregnancy. Some of the exercises that you can do if you have not been following an exercise routine include the following:

- Walking at a brisk pace.
- Swimming in shallow water that is neither too hot nor too cold.
- Pregnancy water workouts.
- Cycling on a stationary cycle or using a step machine at comfortable speed and tension.
- Using a rowing machine at comfortable tension and speed.
- Yoga designed for pregnancy.
- Pelvic toning or kegel exercises.

Well trained pregnant women can also take on these exercises that have been detailed here.

- Cross country skiing.
- Jogging up to about 2 miles per day.
- Doubles tennis (not singles since it can be too strenuous).
- Hiking on plain terrain.
- Dance workouts

Here are some tips that you can use in order to start your workouts:

Warming up is an essential part of exercising and this is something that you must not forget when you are pregnant. Start with 10 minutes of warm--up followed by 5 minutes of strenuous exercise and the 5 minutes of cool down. You can increase the time for the strenuous part after a few days as you become more comfortable.

- Use stretches to ease your muscles. Do not overstretch or bounce, as this is not good for the lax ligaments and muscles.

- Watch the clock at all times and make sure that you do not overdo the exercising in an attempt to remain too fit. Ensure that you do the exercises in moderation to ensure that you are not overdoing the exercises.

- Ensure that you follow a schedule when it comes to the workouts. Being erratic about the exercise schedule may lead to stiffness in the muscles that will take you down to pre-exercising state. If you feel this, then some warm up on the days that you are not able to include a full exercise regime is a good idea.

- Make sure that you consume large amounts of fluids before, during and after the workout.

- Never work out on an empty stomach. Lack of food can make you weak when you are pregnant and this can be extremely risky while working out.

- Wear clothes that are comfortable. The clothes should allow for easy stretch and your underclothes should be made of cotton or those that allow the skin to breathe.

- Exercise on a surface that is wooden or heavily carpeted can help you reduce the impact on your joints. If you are exercising outdoors then you may need to jog on soft running tracks or grassy patches.

It is also recommended that you do not do any exercises that require you to be on your back after the fourth month. Taper of the exercises in the last trimester.

Last but not the least, make sure that you have fun while working out and keep your mood uplifted.

Below are some of the exercises that you can do when you are pregnant.

Over-head Shoulder Stretch

1. Stand with your feet together.

2. Inhale as you lift your right hand overhead; exhale and lean to your left with your left hand on your hip.

3. Hold here as you inhale and exhale five times.

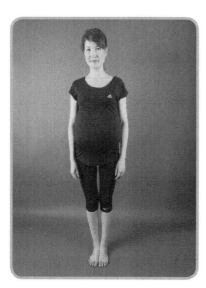
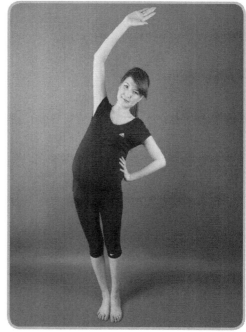

Shoulder Retract

1. Sit upright on a chair and ensure that your back is straight. Do not lean on the back of the chair.

2. Bend your elbows and hold them parallel to the floor.

3. Pull backwards with your shoulders and return to the original position.

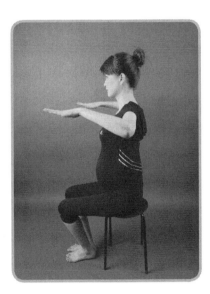
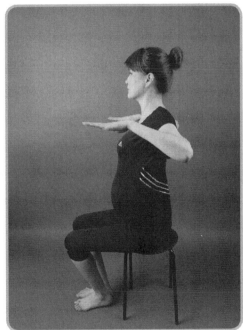

Shoulder Wall Pushups

1. Stand straight with legs at hip distance.

2. Place your hands on the wall.

3. Bend your upper body and try to push the wall. Make sure that you do not bend your legs or move them from the original position.

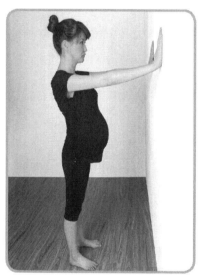
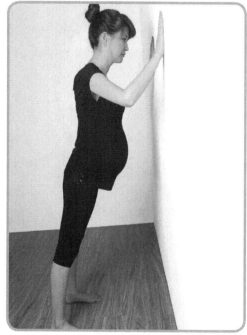

Squat Pose

1. Stand with your feet two to three feet apart, toes pointed out forty five degrees or more.

2. Slowly bend your knees, keeping your spine tall, and glide your hands along your thighs as you sit into a deep squat

3. Your goal is to reach your hands toward the floor while keeping you head above your heart.

4. Hold for 5 breaths.

5. Beginner modification: If you cannot get this deep into the squat, face a wall and glide your hands down along the wall till you are comfortable.

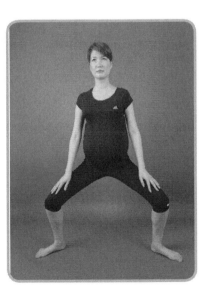
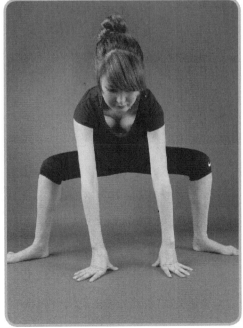

Seated Birth Pose

1. Sit on the floor (if possible) or on your pillow

2. Extend your legs so that they are in a wide V (just outside your hips).

3. Simultaneously bring your knees up towards you.

4. Place your hands on your knees.

5. Gently tug your knees toward your chest, with your feet coming slightly off the floor.

6. Keep your spine aligned and maintain your balance.

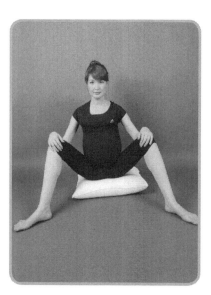
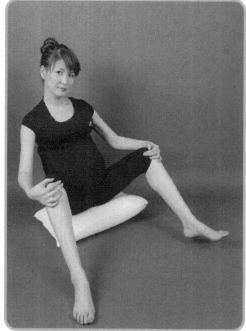

Spinal Flexion With Chair

1. Sit on a chair or couch with your legs spread in a wide V and your arms at your sides.

2. Point your toes to the outside.

3. Gently lower your arms and shoulders between your legs.

4. Rest your hands on the floor just inside your feet.

5. Slowly raise yourself to the starting position.

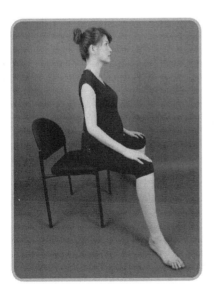
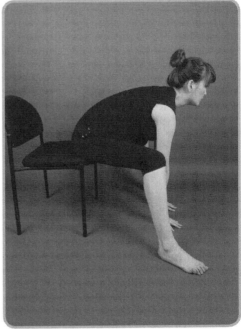

Spinal Extension With Chair Support

1. Kneel in front of an chair with your knees spread in a wide V.

2. Raise your hands over your head as you tilt forward from your waist.

3. Rest your hands on the chair.

4. Keep your head and spine aligned.

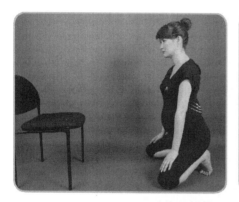
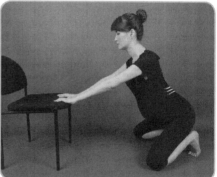
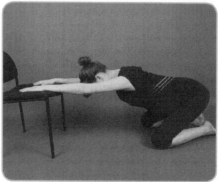

Iso-Pelvic Tilt

1. Lie down flat on the back with arms folded on the chest.

2. Place a pillow under your knees and cross your legs.

3. Lift your waist area and hold it for a few seconds before bringing it down.

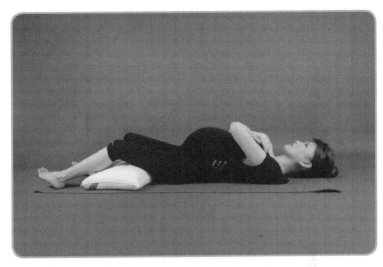

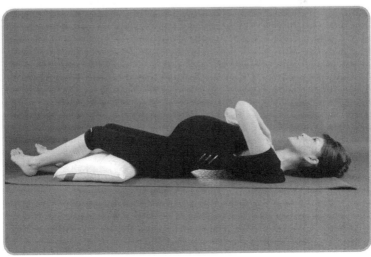

Stretch Hip

1. Sit on the exercise mat and bring the underside of the feet together.

2. Place both your hands below the knees and bring the knees closer together.

3. Hold the position for a few seconds and then return to the original position.

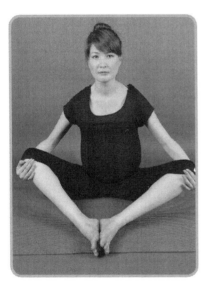
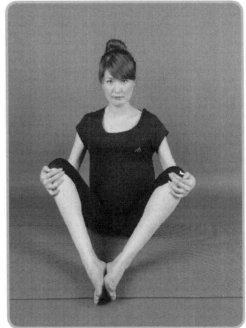

Hip Flex

1. Lie on the floor with one knee bent and the other straight.

2. Lift the straight leg as high as you comfortably can and bring it back to the floor.

3. Repeat the exercise about 20 times and then move on to the next leg.

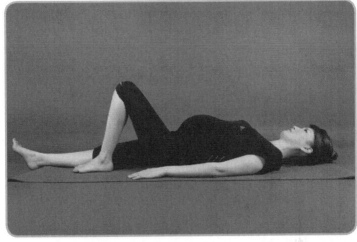

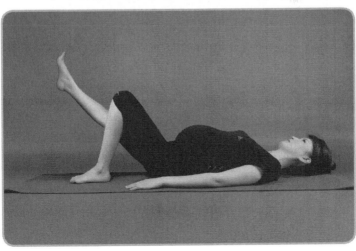

Leg Slide

1. Lie down on your back with hands on the sides.

2. Bend one leg and bring it as close to the hip as you can comfortably.

3. Return to the original position.

4. Continue doing this for about 20 repetitions and the repeat with the other leg.

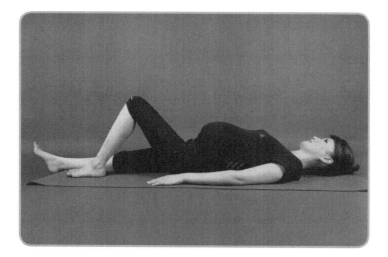

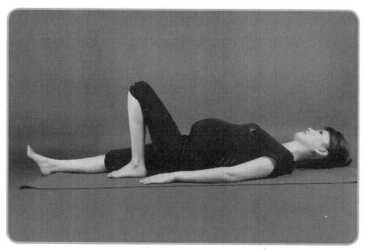

Lumbar Leg Extension

1. The starting position for this exercise is on your knees with your hands on the floor at shoulder width.

2. Lift one leg to make it completely parallel to the body and bring it back to the original position.

3. Continue for 20 repetitions and then do the same with the other leg.

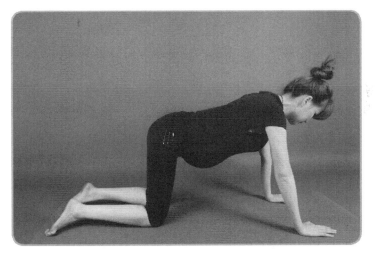

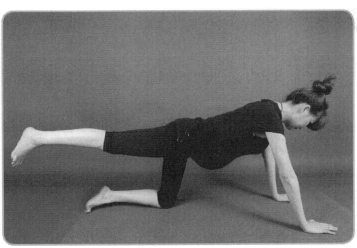

The American College of Obstetricians and Gynecologists lays down certain guidelines as to when you should discontinue exercise. If there are any risk factors that may lead to preterm labor, vaginal bleeding, rupture of membranes prematurely, incompetent cervix, multiple gestation or intrauterine growth retardation, you should refrain yourself from exercises. In case you have hypertension, gestational diabetes, history of premature labor, a respiratory condition, a heart condition, placenta previa or pre-eclampsia, you need to consult your physician before you start exercising.

The guidelines for exercising can also be remembered by using the acronym FITT. This refers to the Frequency, Intensity, Time and Type. Exercise should be done 3 to 5 times a week. The intensity should be moderate. The time should not exceed more than 40 minutes per session and the type of exercise should be low impact, aerobic-type exercise.

The first three months are very important for a pregnancy. If you have been working out prior to pregnancy you can continue to exercise as long as you follow the FITT guidelines. However, if you have not been active prior to getting pregnant, you must avoid exercising for a while. In any case, nausea and vomiting may not allow you to exercise and you need to listen to your body. Using this time, you can easily lie on your back to strengthen your abdominal muscles, since they get weaker as the pregnancy proceeds. It has been seen that women with strong abdominal muscles get back to their pre-pregnancy figure faster than those who have weaker muscles.

From the second trimester onwards, you shall be able to increase the intensity of your workouts by 10 to 15 percent. But continue to listen to your body. Since the ligaments become more elastic due to the hormones, your joints may become looser than before. Avoid any exercises that involve jerky movements or bouncing. The belly that will now start to show slowly also gets you off balance and the center of gravity changes. The strain shifts from the regular joints and ligaments to new ones that may not be so used to the load-bearing. Avoid advanced exercises like push-ups, double leg raises, full sit-ups, jumping, hopping, skipping or any kind of quick dance moves.

Remember that the energy expenditure of a pregnant woman is approximately 300 calories more than a non-pregnant person. If you are also exercising, you need to eat accordingly to make up for the calorie loss that is taking place. Some experts feel that there are chances of hyperthermia in pregnant women who exercise. This is something that can potentially harm the fetus. However, it has been seen that the temperature increase in pregnant women is not as high as it is among those who are not pregnant. This is probably linked with the fact that pregnant women undertake only moderate exercise. Pregnant women who exercise should also take in large amounts of fluids. A pint before exercising and a cup of water after every 20 minutes is recommended.

It should also be noted that when your fetus grows the chances of lumbar lordosis increase. This means that the center of gravity moves towards the pelvis causing an increase in the cervical spine flexion. Some exercises like skiing and tennis should be given up in the third trimester since water retention hinders mobility in the wrists, ankles and can potentially lead to carpel tunnel syndrome.

CHAPTER 13

LABOR AND DELIVERY

The process of labor and delivery is not likely to be an easy one for you with no work on your part. If you have chosen to opt for a caesarean delivery or if you have been told that you need to have one, then you will have a predetermined date when you will arrive at the hospital after full-term and you shall be taken through the specific steps of preparing for the caesarean. On the other hand, if you have started experiencing normal signs of labor, you will need to know about some specific aspects of labor in order to ensure that you are comfortable during the process.

Pain in the Back

For some, back pain can become extremely difficult to handle when labor begins. This is a condition that can happen when the fetus is in the posterior position and the back of the head is pushing against the sacrum or the rear boundary of the pelvis. This is likely to happen to a higher extent for moms who have scoliosis, since the curve in the spine may cause it to form an angle that may result in higher pressure on the spine. It is for this reason that e xperts advise that the management of labor be discussed and pre-planned in consultation with the GP, midwife, obstetrician and the anaesthestist.

Epidural pain relief as an option?

Moreover, here it is also is important to know that though epidural pain relief is an option, yet the epidural insertion might be quite a challenging task for women who either have severe scoliosis or who've had corrective surgery with the help of metal implants and fusion. This is mainly because in such patients, it is quite difficult to locate the right point for administering the local anesthetic.
It is for such reasons that other pain relief options be analyzed. In fact, it is always better to inform the obstetric anesthetist of any such medical history so that suitable options can be decided in advance.

The bad news is that this kind of pain does not let up between contractions. The good news is that it is not an indication of a problem and is likely to end when delivery is over. There are some steps you can take in order to relieve yourself of the pain.

Change your position now and then and reduce the amount of pressure that you are putting on your back. Try walking around if you think you can, crouch or squat. Getting down on all fours is also an option that takes the pressure off the back immensely. If you feel that you cannot get off the bed, then try to change your position and move on to your side for a while.

Using a heat compress or hot water bottle is a great idea too, but some people may feel that a cold compress works better. Alternately, you can also use a hot compress followed by a cold compress and then a hot compress again. Ask your partner or the person who is accompanying you to put counter pressure on to the area where it hurts the most. Circular motion or the use of knuckles works well. Acupressure has also been used to relieve pain. For back labor pain, you will need to ask someone to apply pressure below the center of the ball of the foot. This needs to be done with an appreciable force with a finger.

Labor Positions

The amount of pain that you are likely to go through during labor makes you feel that you just want to lie down on your back. However, this is the one position that you should not spend your labor period in. What then, you may ask, is the best position to adopt? The best position is the one that you feel most comfortable in, other than on your back.

The back position is not recommended because it puts a large amount of pressure on your back; something that can cause a lot of strain. It also slows down the labor process making you go through labor for a much longer time than necessary. It compresses some of the major blood vessels and therefore interferes with the flow of blood to the fetus.

An upright position will help with the force of gravity working along with your contractions to push the baby out. Standing, sitting in bed, squatting, kneeling and even straddling a chair are options that can be chosen. If you feel you have to lie down, then try lying down on your left side.

Stages of labor

There are, in fact, three stages of labor that have been defined. How quickly you move from one stage to another is something that cannot be determined by anyone.

The three stages of labor include latent, active and transitional. These are parts of the first phase of delivery that is called labor. In the first stage of labor, there is a thinning of the cervix that happens along with a dilation of the cervix to about 3 centimeters. In the second stage the dilation is more active and the cervix dilates till about 7 centimeters. In the third stage the dilation reaches its maximum of 10 centimeters, indicating that you are at the peak of labor and it is time to go into the delivery room.

All women go through these phases unless it is cut short by a need to do a caesarian. Sometimes, you may not even realize that you have entered labor until you are in the second or even third stage of the process. This can happen if the contractions in the first and second phase are relatively less intense.

Pain and Perception

Pain is a relatively subjective phenomenon and it can be heightened and alleviated by several factors. It may surprise you to know that the perception of pain is something that you can control to a large extent. Some of the factors that increases the perception of pain include being alone, feeling tired, hunger and thirst, continuously thinking about pain, stress and exerting during contractions, fear of the unknown aspect of delivery and feeling self-pity and helpless.

On the other hand, there are aspects that can help you decrease the perception of pain. These include having someone you love close by, being relaxed, ensuring that you do not starve completely during labor, distracting yourself from the pain and thinking of something else, using relaxation techniques like meditation, visualization and learning everything you can about labor.

Stages of Childbirth

The entire process of childbirth has three phases. The first is labor that you have already read. The second is the pushing stage where the actual delivery of the baby happens and the third is the removal of the placenta.

During the labor stage, you need to ensure that you are as comfortable as you can be with the contractions. Try to listen to some music. If you are lucky to have a television in your labor room then you can distract yourself from the pain by watching something interesting. Sip on water or orange juice and eat a light snack whenever you feel hunger pangs. Staying hungry will only make you feel more tired and fatigued. Time your contractions in between to know whether it is time to rush to the hospital or not. As you progress into the second stage of labor, you should start doing your breathing exercises. Try to relax between the contractions and urinate frequently even if you feel that you do not need to. The last part of the labor, just before you get into the delivery phase is likely to be tough. The contractions will come much faster and will be more intense. Remain positive and think of the fact that you are almost there now and that the task at hand cannot last much longer.

The delivery phase is where you will need to do a lot of hard work. Once the dilation has reached the level where you can get into labor, you will need to do some active pushing. At this stage, you may have a strong urge to push and may experience some renewed levels of energy. On the other hand, you could also feel extremely fatigued and may want it all to "just end". There is also likely to be a tingling, stretching and burning sensation in the vaginal area as the head of the baby starts appearing. If you push more efficiently, you can be sure that the ordeal will last for much lesser time. The idea is to push from the part of your body that is below the navel since pushing from the chest can cause chest pain after the delivery. Follow the instructions of your practitioner, because he or she will be able to tell you the exact time when the pushing will help the most.

When you are pushing at this stage, you should not think much of passing stuff that is in your rectum or passing urine inadvertently. This is not something that you should be concerned about because it happens in many cases and your doctors too are not likely to think about it even once. Take your breaks when the doctor asks you to relax and build up all your energy to start pushing again.

The third stage of the delivery is also necessary. At this point, you have brought your baby into this world efficiently and safely. Though there is still some work to be done. The placenta that has been helping your baby live within you also needs to be delivered. Mild contractions may continue. Check with the doctor as you need to help deliver the placenta by pushing. After the placenta is delivered, the doctor will sew up if an episiotomy had been necessary. You could now relax and enjoy your baby!

Caesarean Delivery

If you are having a caesarean delivery, the level of your involvement is likely to be much lower. In fact, all you need to do is be mentally and physically prepared for the surgery and leave the rest in the able hands of the surgeons. It is likely that your abdomen will be shaved and washed with antiseptic solution. A catheter may also be inserted into the bladder so that it does not interfere with the approach to your uterus.

In most cases, you will be given an epidural anesthesia and you are not likely to feel anything from the waist down in a few minutes. This is not likely to knock you out completely and therefore you shall be able to see the process if you have requested a mirror or screen. A horizontal incision is made just above the bikini line and the recti muscles are retracted away from the midline. The bladder is protected by retracting it downwards. The uterus is opened at the lower margin and the amniotic fluid sac is ruptured, if it already has not ruptured on its own. The liquid is suctioned out and baby is eased out. The cord is then clamped and cut and the nose and the mouth of the baby are suctioned to enable the baby to start breathing.

You will be stitched up after delivery. In some cases, surgeons prefer to give a short general anesthetic to the mother at this time to allow her to relax. This lasts for less than 30 minutes and by the time you are stitched up and moved out into the recovery room, your baby shall be washed and cleaned and brought to your side as well.

Epidural Anesthesia

An epidural is also an option for pain-relief, even if you are not having a Caesarean delivery. This regional anesthesia blocks the pain in the abdominal and the vaginal region. Sometimes, an epidural is used with epinephrine, fentanyl, morphine or clonidine to increase the effect or manage blood pressure. The epidural injection is given before active labor begins. It can be given while you are lying on your left side or sitting up; in both cases with your back arched.

There are two main types of epidurals – regular and combined spinal-epidural. The regular epidural is a combination of narcotics and anesthesia that is administered through a pump or periodic injections. The latter is also called the 'walking epidural' since it allows you to move about more freely.

An epidural can help you relax if the labor is exceptionally painful or if it prolongs for a long period of time. The relief from pain also allows you to be an active participant in the birth process. Sometimes, epidural injections may cause some shivering, headaches or temporary tinnitus but these disadvantages are insignificant in comparison to the relief that it provides.

The process of injecting an epidural does not hurt. There is also no research that has shown any negative effects on the baby. While you may not be able to feel the contractions due to the numbing effect, you shall be able to push on cue by your doctor. Some aid may be required in terms of pushing the abdomen in order to help the process.

Sometimes the anesthesiologist may not be able to find the epidural space due to your scoliosis condition. This is something that can happen among those who do not have scoliosis too, if they have back problems or excessive weight gain. Given your condition, you should prepare for a delivery without an epidural in case it becomes difficult in your case to find the epidural space. Check out other pain relief methods like massage, positioning and Transcutaneous Electrical Nerve Stimulation (TENS).

CHAPTER 14

POST NATAL EXERCISES FOR WOMEN WITH SCOLIOSIS

Post natal exercises are extremely important for all women. These exercises can not only help you regain your pre-pregnancy shape but they can also help in ensuring that your body gets back the strength it has lost in the process of pregnancy and childbirth. The exercises make your body strong and allow the muscles and ligaments to gain their previous health, strength and energy. Once you have gained some level of comfort with these exercises, you can then shift to doing exercises that are tailored towards straightening the abnormal spinal curve, explained in my previous book 'Your Plan for Natural Scoliosis Prevention and Treatment, Health in Your Hands'.

However, there are a lot of things that you need to keep in mind when you are getting back to exercising after childbirth. Do not make the mistake of being in too much of a hurry to get your shape back because it can do much larger damages to your weak muscles. Remember that there are a lot of after-effects of childbirth that need to settle down before you start your regular routine. Make use of this time to bond with your child and spend as much time as you can with the baby.

Tips to Adhere to before Starting Post Natal Exercises

It is important that you have a post-natal checkup before your return to exercising in a big way. This is something you can opt for after 6 weeks of delivery. Those who have had a caesarean delivery may have to wait for about 8 to 10 weeks after delivery to start exercising. The reason that makes it necessary to wait for a few weeks before exercising is the lingering effect of relaxin that leads to relaxed ligaments and lose abdominal muscles. The few weeks after delivery are critical to allow the uterus to shrink back to its normal size and to ensure that bleeding ceases. In case there are stitches in the vaginal area, these need to heal as well.

When you start exercising after your post-natal checkup, make sure that you are well prepared for the sessions. Here are some tips that you will find useful in order to be fully prepared for your exercising sessions post-delivery.

- Make sure that the clothing that you choose is extremely comfortable so that it allows easy movement. Some women prefer loose clothing especially at the pelvic and spinal area. However, make sure that your trainer can see your posture in order to correct it if the form is wrong while you are exercising. The bra that you use should fit well so that there is no excessive squeezing of the breasts. On the other hand, the bra should not be too loose to allow for excessive bouncing; something that can be extremely uncomfortable. You may also want to use breast pads in case you feel that you are likely to have a leakage.

- Proper footwear is also necessary in order to ensure that the impact that transmits through the spine is minimal. The shoes that you choose should have proper shock absorption capabilities.

- Make sure that you never exercise on an empty stomach. While you may have gone for your gym sessions early in the morning pre-pregnancy, this is not the time to continue the old routine. Eat something a couple of hours before the activity so that you have the energy to perform the exercises well. Packing in a light carbohydrate meal 30 minutes before the exercising session is also a good idea. You can also eat about 15 minutes after the exercise to allow for better absorption and digestion of the carbohydrates.

- Finding time for a 2-hour exercise session may not be possible with pending household chores to catch-up on when the baby is sleeping. In addition to that, there are days when you will need to catch-up on your own sleep due to a sleepless night as well. Do not try to achieve too much in a little time. Try to squeeze multiple small exercising sessions at home in case you cannot get 2 hours flat for the workout.

- It is not appropriate to do resistance exercises when you are tired. However, light exercises of the right intensity can actually make you feel more energetic and lively. A walk, with the baby in the buggy, in the fresh air can help you feel better.

- It is very easy to start overdoing things when you have been used to a good shape prior to pregnancy. Some women are extremely eager to get back to their old shape as soon as possible and they end up overdoing the exercise sessions. Remember that lack of cautiousness in this area can lead to issues later that may have more significant consequences.

- Watch out for the warning signs that will tell you to take a break from exercising. Breathlessness, dizziness and nausea are the key signs. If you feel that you are getting clumsy on the cardiovascular machine or find difficulty in motor coordination, it is advisable to stop for a while. Trembling muscles and holding breath after a few repetitions is also something that you should look out for.

Reactivation of Transversus Abdominis muscle (TrA)

The reactivation of the TrA is the first exercise that you should undertake after you leave the hospital. TrA is a postural muscle that maintains lumbo-pelvic stability along with other local stabilizers. This is a muscle that needs to be reactivated post-delivery since the pregnancy has realigned the muscles that are being used for stability.

There are some simple steps that can be used to activate TrA.

- Stand or sit upright and place your fingers on the hip bone at the front.

- Move your fingers diagonally into the soft tissue of the abdomen.

- Apply some pressure on the soft tissue and cough lightly.

- At this time you will feel the TrA and Internal Oblique (IO) contract.

- You can also achieve the same effect without coughing and by pulling the abdomen in.

Following these simple steps is all that you need in order to activate the TrA. In addition to locating the TrA, it is also necessary that you learn to adopt the proper stance while exercising and learning to breathe properly while exercising.

Post-natal Exercises

Post-natal exercises can be divided into various categories. These include stretching exercises, mobilization exercises and stabilization exercises. While resistance and strength training are also types of exercises that you can do, these should be limited due to the excessive laxity in the muscles and ligaments. The relaxed muscular environment can cause the skeletal structure to be compromised if these exercises are done before complete recovery is achieved.

Below I have discussed some mobilization, stretching and stability exercises that you can start after delivery.

Mobilization exercises

Mobilization exercises are the ones that you should start with initially. This is because these are light exercises that loosen the body and provide the flexibility that is required to do the other exercises. It is recommended that you go back to the most basic exercises when you have been given the go ahead from your physician after the post-natal checkup. This is important and essential even if you have been doing more advanced exercises before you got pregnant.

It is very likely that your standing stance is wider than it should be. This happens because you are likely to feel that your hips have widened. Make special note of this and ensure that you keep your feet as wide as your hips and not more.

Below are some of the mobilization exercises that you should start with.

Shoulder Circle

1. The idea of the shoulder circle is to mobilize the shoulder joint.

2. You need to stand in the right standing posture with the arms on the side in a relaxed position.

3. Draw in the abdomen and then move the shoulder in a circular manner. Make sure that you move it forward, upwards, backwards and then downwards. Repeat this movement a 20 times on both sides.

4. Make sure that your knees are slightly bent; the stance is upright and maintain slow and controlled movement of the shoulder.

5. Repeat the set of exercises by moving the shoulder backward, upward, forward and then downwards.

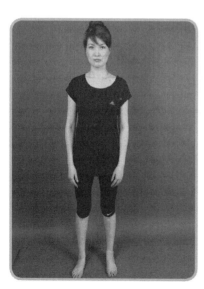
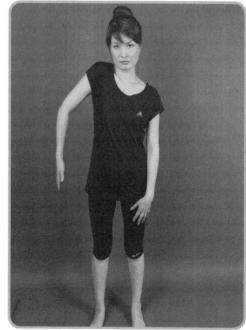

Side Bend

1. This exercise helps in increasing the mobility of the spine.

2. The posture of standing in the upright position with the hands in a relaxed position on the sides is to be maintained. Make sure that the feet are not too wide as this can cause the hips to sway during the exercises; something that causes lateral spinal flexion.

3. Draw the abdomen in and bend sideways. Make sure that the movement is from the waist. Bend only as much as you can comfortably without trying to stretch too much.

4. Return to the original position and repeat on the other side.

5. Repeat this movement a 20 times on both sides.

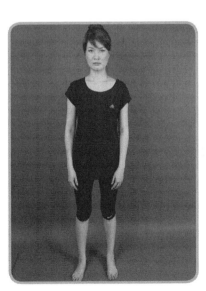 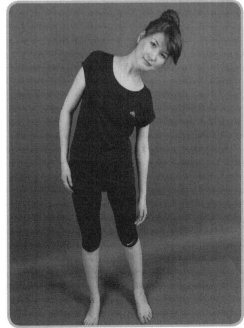

Trunk Rotation

1. Trunk rotation helps in mobilization of the thoracic spine; a part that becomes stiff during pregnancy.

2. For this exercise, you need to stand in the upright position and bend the elbows and lift them to the height of the chest.

3. Keeping the abdomen drawn in, rotate the upper body to one side.

4. Return to the original position and then turn to the other side.

5. Keep the shoulder blades downwards and try to lengthen the spine as you rotate the upper body. Make sure that the hips and knees are not used for rotating.

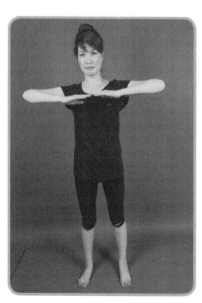
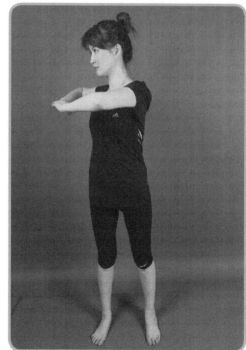

Hip Rotation

1. The main aim of hip rotation is to loosen the lower back.

2. You need to stand in the upright position and place hands at the lower rib-cage level with the elbows bent.

3. Draw the abdomen in and move the hips in an extended circle. Make sure that the knees are slightly bent and spine long.

4. Try to ensure that the movement that occurs is mainly below the waist and that the upper body does not move. The chest should remain lifted while trying to get the full range of rotation possible comfortably.

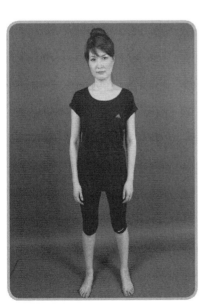
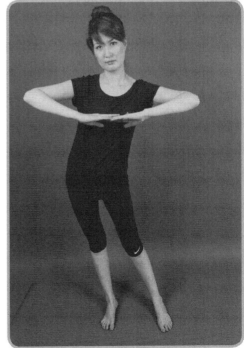

Trunk Curl

1. This is an exercise that you should do to ensure loosening of the upper body and to open up the chest.

2. You need to stand in upright position, the arms must be held outwards towards the sides.

3. Keep the abdominal muscles pulled in and then tilt the pelvis by curling the tailbone.

4. Round the upper part of the body and as you do so move the arms inwards towards the front of the body.

5. Return to the original position and move the arms sideways too.

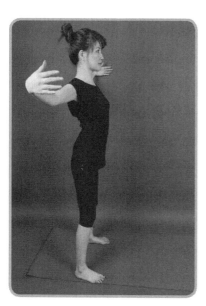
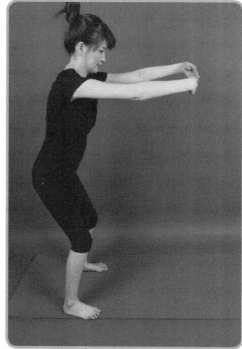

Neck Mobility

1. This is an exercise that helps in reducing tension in the neck.

2. The initial stance of this exercise is to stand upright with the arms on the sides.

3. With the abdominal muscles tucked in, turn the head in order to look over the shoulder.

4. Stop for a second and then return to the center and then repeat on the other side.

5. Make sure that you do not tip your head to the side and lengthen the spine every time you return to the original position.

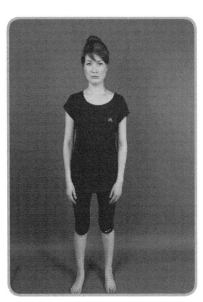
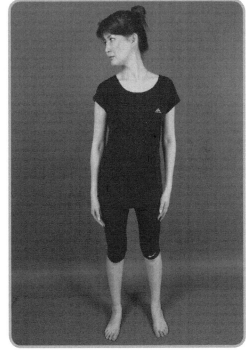

Stretching exercises

The spine goes through a lot of stress through the nine months that you carry the baby. There is a significant amount of muscle tightness that develops through the spine due to the different postures that one needs to adopt in order to carry the baby and for the later care of the baby too. Make sure that you do not hold the stretches for more than 15 to 30 seconds, since you do not want to harm the muscles that are still too lax.

Here are some stretching exercises that you can benefit from after you have delivered and completed the post-natal checkup.

Rainbow Stretch

1. This is a stretching exercise that works on the thoracic spine and it stretches the pectoral muscles too.

2. The starting position of this exercise is to lie on the floor sideways with a pillow under the head. Both the hands need to be extended and joined together as in a prayer and rested on the floor. The knees also need to be bent and joined together.

3. While pulling in the abdominal muscles, the upper arm should be lifted to the ceiling. At the same time turn the head upwards to look at the ceiling.

4. Move the hand to the other side and make sure to follow the hand movement with the head movement.

5. Once the arm reaches the other side, pause for a while and breathe.

6. Use the abdominal muscles to pull back the hand to the original position.

7. Make sure that the pelvic and the lumbar areas of the spine remain in the original position.

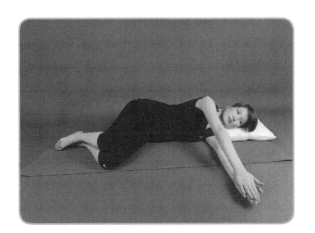

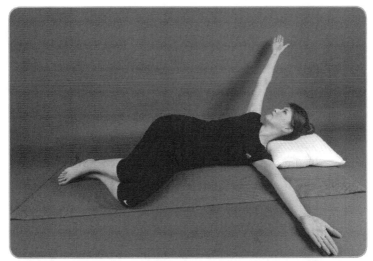

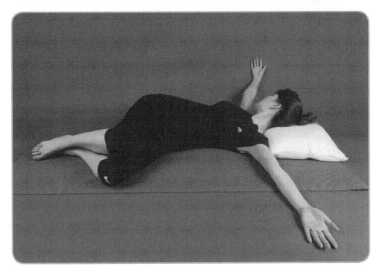

Seated Pectoral Stretch

1. This exercise helps in improving the posture and in lengthening pectoral muscles.

2. It can be done by sitting on the floor in an upright posture with legs in a criss-cross position.

3. Make sure that you sit up straight and take your hands backwards and place them on the floor. This should be done without leaning backwards in any way.

4. Draw in the abdomen, open the chest and draw the elbows backwards.

5. You will feel the chest and the shoulders stretching at this stage.

6. It is important that you open the chest and not lift it if you want the stretch to have proper effect.

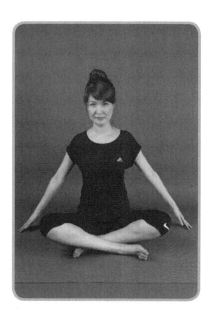 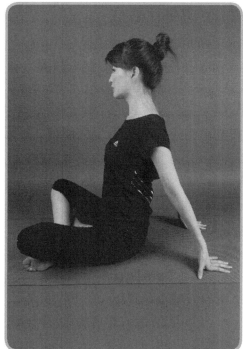

Seated Trapeze Stretch

1. The idea of this exercise is to reduce the stress in the mid-trapezius muscles with postural changes.

2. While sitting on the floor in an upright position, the arms need to be extended outwards towards the sides.

3. The shoulder blades should be down.

4. As you tilt the pelvic bone upwards, the arms need to be brought in and the spine needs to be curved in along with the head.

5. Catch hold of the elbow of the opposite arm and make the shoulder lean and press forward.

6. Natural breathing should continue at all times during this stretch.

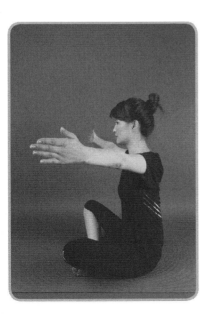
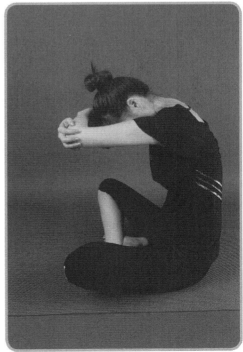

Seated Latissimus Dorsi Stretch

1. This is an exercise that lessens the ache and stress in the latissimus dorsi and helps in better thoracic mobility.

2. Sit on the floor in an upright position and rest the tips of the hands on the floor on the sides. This should be slightly in front of the hips.

3. Lift one hand and take it upwards as if you were trying to touch the ceiling. Feel the stretch on the side of the hand that you have lifted.

4. Continue moving in an arch while moving the hand on the floor further away from the body.

5. Move backwards into the original position.

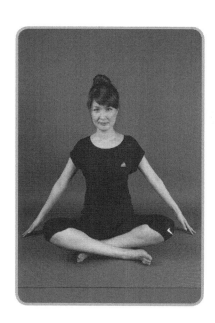 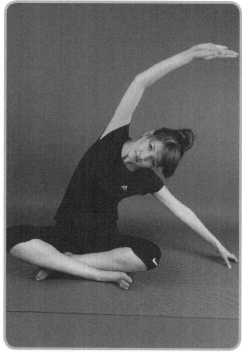

Seated Neck Stretch

1. This exercise helps in lessening the tension in the neck muscles.

2. The starting position is upright posture on the floor with hands on the sides.

3. Tilt the head to one side and take the ear to the shoulder. Make sure that you do not raise the shoulder to try to meet the ear.

4. Bring back to original position and move towards the other side.

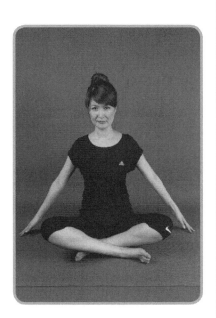 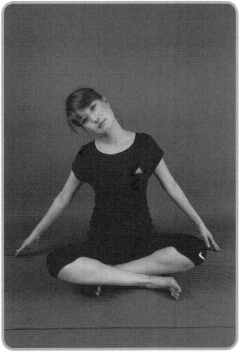

Standing Upward Reach

1. This is one exercise that brings great refreshment.

2. You need to stand in a straight position and keep your arms on the side in a relaxed manner.

3. Take a deep breath and then move your arms upwards and outwards towards the ceiling. Feel the spine lengthening.

4. Exhale as you bring the arms down.

5. Make sure to draw the shoulder blades down as the arms lift up. Keep your arms slightly forward to maintain the neutral stance.

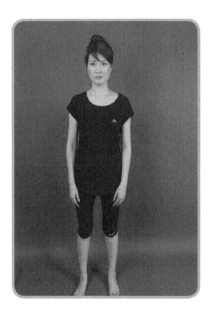
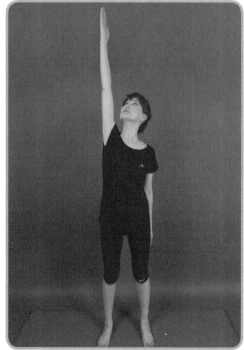

Standing Side Stretch

1. Use this stretch to lengthen the latissimus dorsi muscles and to release the tension in them. This exercise also helps in increasing thoracic mobility.

2. The start of this exercise is to stand in the upright position with the hands on the hips.

3. Pull in the abdominal muscles and reach out to the ceiling with one hand and then continue to move the hand towards the other side stretching the side of the waist.

4. If you are lifting the right arm, you should feel a stretch in the right side of your body.

5. Bring the arm back and lower the hand and repeat.

6. Repeat with the other hand too.

7. Do not push the hip to the other side and do not bend the other side as well.

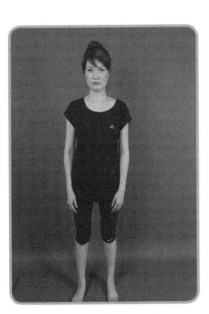
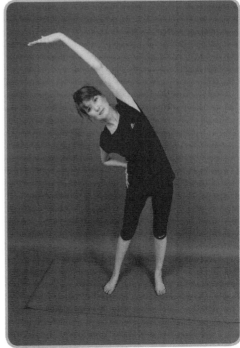

Beginner Core Stabilization Exercises

Stabilization exercises are great for the new mom. A stability ball should be used in order to strengthen the core abdominal muscles that have weakened considerably through the pregnancy period. Your core is essentially the center of your body – more specifically, your abdominal muscles and the muscles of the hips, butt, back, and pelvic floor. All of your core muscles work together as a unit; they are all connected by fascia, a layer of connective tissue.

Here are some core exercises that you can benefit from after you have delivered and which are essential in your quest for a flat stomach.

Pelvic Floor Warm-Up

1. Lie on your back with the crook of your knees bent. There will be a space between the floor and your lower back, as well as your neck. This because your core is not activated yet.

2. Inhale, and as you exhale, tilt your pelvis toward your belly button. It is a small move and you will not really see much movement in your tummy. Continue to pull without letting your stomach "pooch out."

3. Hold this position as long as is comfortable, up to 10 seconds, then rest for 10 seconds

4. Relax your pelvic floor.

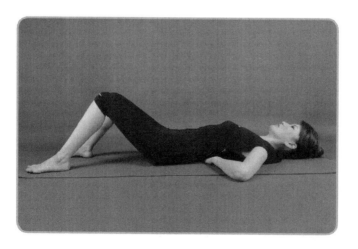

Four-Point Tummy Vacuum

1. Kneel down with your hips over your knees and your shoulders over the palm of your hands

2. With your spine in a comfortable position without stress in a neutral alignment, take a deep breath in and let your stomach drop toward the floor.

3. Breathe out and draw your navel in toward your spine, while keeping your back in the starting position

4. Hold for as long as you comfortably can

5. When you need to breathe in, relax your abdominal wall as you inhale and repeat the exercise 10 times

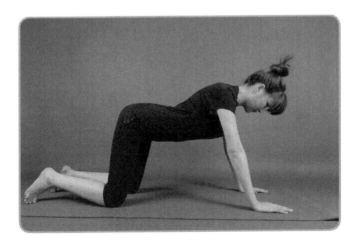

Plank Position

1. Start by lying face down on the ground or use an exercise mat. Place your elbows and forearms underneath your chest

2. Prop yourself up to form a bridge using your toes and forearms.

3. Maintain a flat back and do not allow your hips to sag towards the ground.

4. Hold for 60 seconds

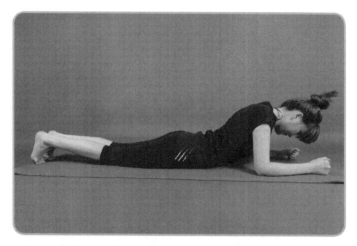

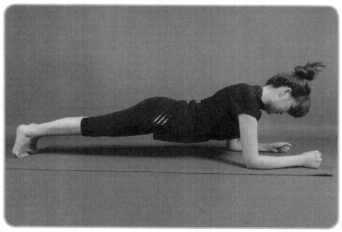

Lunge Core Twist

1. From a standing position with feet together, clasp your hands, with straight arms at shoulder height, to your left.

2. Step forward and lunge with your right leg, rotate from the waist, and twist to the right.

3. Then step forward and lunge with your left leg, rotate from the waist, and twist to the left.

4. Repeat 20 times.

5. To make it harder, use 3-8 pound weights.

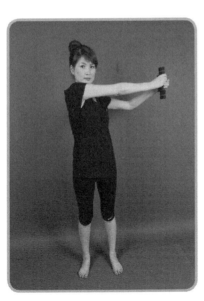
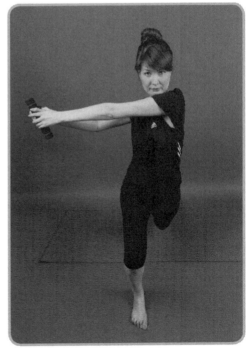

Caution if You Have Had a C-Section

The exercises mentioned in this book are safe and easy to do. However, if you have had a C-section some of these may irritate the incision area. If you feel even the slightest of discomfort, take a break for some time till you are completely fine with starting again. It is also a great idea to support your abdominal area with the help of a pillow for better comfort.

In most cases you shall be able to start exercising about 6 weeks after delivery. Those who have had a vaginal delivery can start earlier. You might also feel numbness for some time after the procedure. Remember that your nerves were cut as well during the C-Section and these will take time to recover.

The Shelf After a C-Section

Many women worry about the shelf that forms over the C-Section scar. However, you can get rid of the shelf too if you work out and make your muscles work for you. Dr. Kent Snowden, Obstetrician and gynecologist states that 'the shelf is most likely fatty tissue damage'. Once the swelling is down and you are back to normal life, the only memory of the C-section will probably be the scar tissue. However, make sure that you give this at least 6 months.

Advanced Core Stabilization Exercises

Once you have comfortably completed the beginner core stabilisation exercises its time to move on to the advanced core stability exercises that target different areas of your core.

Forward Ball Roll

1. Kneel in front of a Swiss ball with your forearms just behind the highest point of the ball. The angle at your hips and shoulders should be the same. Imagine being able to place a box in between the back of your arms and thighs

2. Gently draw the navel inward and hold a good comfortable position of your back and head

3. Roll forward, moving your legs and arms in equal measure so that the angles at the shoulders and hips remain equal, as you roll farther away. Progressively increase the effort used to draw your navel inward

4. Stop at the point just before you lose form. You will feel your lower back drop down when your form breaks. You should stop just before this point

5. For beginners, go to the finish position and hold for three seconds, then return to the start position. Your tempos should be three seconds out, three seconds hold, three seconds return.

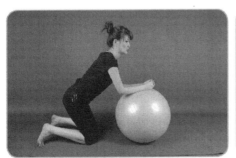 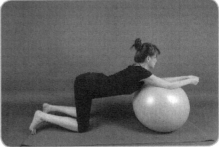

Swiss Ball Crunch

Caution: If you get dizzy while performing this exercise, you can lean a little forward on the ball. In any case, stop this exercise immediately if you continue to feel dizzy

1. Lie over a Swiss ball so that your back is comfortably rested on the ball.

2. Keep your tongue against the roof of your mouth

3. As you slowly crunch up, imagine that you are rolling your spine from head to pelvis

4. On the way back, unwind from the lower back to your head, one vertebra at a time

5. Breathe out on the way up and inhale on the way back

6. Arm positioning

   Beginner — arms stretched out and reaching forward
   Intermediate — arms kept across chest
   Advanced — finger tips behind ears (do not support your head and neck with your hands)

7. Tempo should be slow, breathing pace.

8. Repeat 20 times.

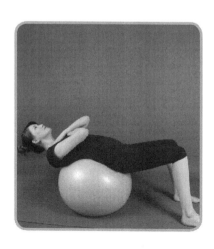
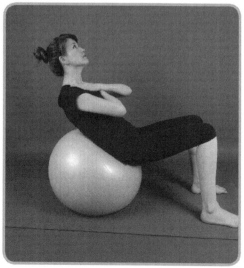

Dynamic Horse Stance

1. Get on your hands and knees with your wrist directly under the shoulders and knees directly under the hips

2. Contract the abdominals and slowly straighten your right leg behind you, turning your foot slightly out while extending your left arm in front of you, thumb up

3. Repeat on one side for a set of 10

4. Release and repeat with left leg and right arm

In addition to the stretching, mobilizing and stabilizing exercises, a water work out is a great thing to practice even after delivery. It is most likely that you have been using water exercises during your pregnancy and if you have enjoyed these then you should make it a point to continue it after delivery too.

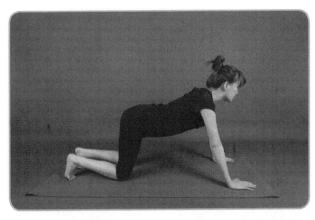

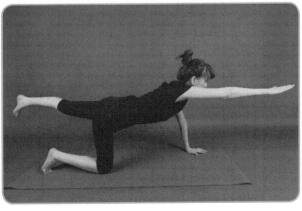

Water workouts

There are various benefits of exercising in water. For one there is a much lesser amount of stress that the joints have to tolerate. It is also easier to work out in the water when you have gained weight. The water pressure that exerts itself on various parts of the body is good for blood circulation too. The good circulation obtained also helps in moving the blood effectively through the kidneys so that water retention, that is an integral part of the weight gain during pregnancy, can be reduced. The hydrostatic pressure also helps in forcing the retained fluids from the tissues into the circulation. It has also been seen that the after-effects of exercise done in water are not felt as much as those done on land. You are, therefore, less likely to feel soreness in the muscles. And last but not the least, the water has a therapeutic effect that calms you down. It helps you gain composure and relaxes you to a large extent.

Additionally, the water slows down the movements that you carry out. This means that if you are someone who has been used to high impact and quick reflex exercises, you will be able to manage the situation better. Water exercises are a great way in which you can do some of the exercises that you otherwise find tough. This is mainly because of the lower amount of gravity that you experience in the water.

When you choose a water workout, you need to remember that the resistance of water is much higher than that of air. Therefore walking or moving upright is likely to take much more effort than on land. The resistance is also present in all directions. Group sessions create turbulence that increases the amount of resistance.

Make sure that the temperature of the water in the pool is around 20 degrees Celsius. Warmer water is likely to increase the elasticity of the muscles, something that you do not want. Warm water can also encourage milk secretion. Cold water can constrict blood vessels leading to poor circulation while you are exercising. The height of the pool should be approximately till the chest level. This will support the pelvic floor, the chest and the breasts. This depth of the pool will also help you in ensuring that you can do a good upper body workout in water. You can start on water workouts as soon as the vaginal discharge stops. This is generally sometime between 3 to 5 weeks after delivery.

Among other workouts that you do in the water, swimming is also a great post-natal workout. It helps in increasing cardiovascular ability and provides muscular benefits as well. Start with a few laps where you swim in a relaxed manner and then move to moderately paced swimming for a long time. Try to use the freestyle stroke and avoid any prone stroke that requires you to keep the head high.

Rest and relaxation

While you may be extremely conscious and worried about getting back into shape, it is important to remember that you need to get adequate rest too. Even if you are not used to taking long breaks or naps in the day time, you need to make sure that you feel relaxed during the day. This is something that is good for you and your baby. A happy mom can provide much better care for her baby than an unhappy one.

The baby's arrival is likely to put a lot of pressure on you as a person. This is likely to be much more than you thought possible and definitely much more than what you experienced during the nine months of pregnancy.

Stress is one of the most common aspects that a new mom needs to think about. It is a threat to the body, the well-being of the child and the relationship with the partner as well. When stress strikes, the body starts to save up on all the internal functions that it performs and limits them to a minimum of what is necessary to keep alive. Aspects like digestion, toxin removal and effective breathing are compromised. The idea is to divert all the energy towards fighting off the cause of stress. Unfortunately, while this worked in the ancient times when stress was caused mainly due to physical threats, today the stress generators are generally emotional in nature. But, the body reacts in a similar manner.

If the reaction of the body continues for a long period of time it causes chronic stress and severely compromises the manner in which your body functions.

There are various stress factors that have been associated with post-natal stress. These are either physical or emotional in nature. The physical factors include fatigue, lack of sleep, sore perineum, constipation, joint pain, reduced energy levels, sore and heavy breasts and postural changes. Some of the emotional stress generators include issues with the baby, like crying for a long time, inability to settle the baby, lack of time, feeling of inadequacy as a mother, feeling of isolation and being alone in this fight to manage the child and inability to lose weight quickly.

The body's reaction towards stress includes bent head and body, elevated shoulders, bent elbows close to the body, clenched fists, tight jaws and clenched teeth. The heart rate generally increases during stress and the blood pressure and breathing rate also increase.

It is important that you cope with stress, in order to be able to get your body working normally. There are various methods of relaxation that you can practice. But, it is necessary that you are dedicated towards the cause and believe that stress can not only harm your body but it can also do a lot of harm to your baby indirectly. So make sure that you take out the time to relax and practice some relaxation techniques in order to be calmer and at peace.

The three methods of relaxation that are commonly used are:

- *Contrast methods* — This is a method in which you contract and then relax all large muscles of the body one by one and consciously. You can start by lying down and relaxing and then thinking about one muscle and contracting it. Hold it for a while and then let go. Start from the toe and work all the way up to the shoulders and face. While this is an easy method to follow for relaxation, it may become difficult for people to contract or relax muscles that are already too tense.

- *Visualization* — Also called imagery, this is a method in which you need to ensure that you are in a quiet room with no noise. Close your eyes and start to visualize specific happy images in your mind. This is a psychological exercise but you will realize that it has a direct impact on the way in which you feel when you are done with it.

- *Physiological relaxation* — This method is also called the Mitchell Method and involves reciprocal inhibition. In this method one muscle must be allowed to relax as the other one is contracted. In this method, you need to go through the entire body in a fixed routine.

  - Start with the shoulders and pull them up towards the ears. Be cognizant of the fact that the neck is being elongated.

  - Move the elbows away from the body slowly.

  - Stretch the fingers and feel them being stretched.

  - Roll the hips outwards but keeping the legs slightly apart.

  - Move the knees to a more comfortable position.

  - Flex the toes by bringing them towards the face.

  - Press your body into the bed or mattress that you are lying on.

  - Press the head into the pillow.

  - While ensuring that the lips are together, pull the jaw down.

  - Move the tongue to the middle of the mouth.

  - Close the eyes and be aware of the darkness that it causes.

  - Raise the eyebrows towards the hairline.

  - Take a deep breath and pull in as much air as you can and breathe out slowly.

Once you have completed this session, do so slowly and deliberately.

It is important that when you take out time to relax, you are in appropriate and comfortable gear. It is important that you are in a place where you cannot hear the cries of the baby (this means that you ensure that someone else is looking after your baby for a while or that you have a baby monitor with you if she is sleeping). Try to stop thinking about the chores that you need to complete and the things that you need to achieve before the end of the day. This is not the time that you have put aside for planning your day or your week or your life.

Lifestyle changes

Other than the exercises that you do, a large number of specific chores have probably been added to your life with the arrival of the baby. There are specific movements that you will be adopting in order to hold the baby, feed the baby and even play with the baby. In addition to that it is recommended that some of the regular things that you did earlier should be done properly, in order to avoid any kind of jerky movements that may cause harm.

Here are some tips about the lifestyle changes that you should make post-delivery.

- Sit on the edge of the bed and then rise from it slowly. Keep the knees and legs aligned with getting out so that there is minimal effort.

- Holding the baby on one side is something that many women prefer, this way, they can change the side when they get tired too. There is a tendency to arch the hip slightly to be able to allow for the baby to rest on the protrusion. Such a position is likely to cause a large amount of pressure on the lumbar spine if this holding position has been continued for long.

- Make sure that you are not sitting in a slumped position when you are feeding the baby. Try to get a feeding chair so that you are always upright. Place cushions or a stool underneath your feet if they do not touch the ground easily and comfortably.

- Do not lift the entire baby bath when it is full of water. Choose a baby bath option that you can place within the larger bath so that there are no issues in draining the water.

- Having a changing table for the baby that is waist high for you so that you can work easily. If this is not available, kneel on the side of the bed while changing the baby.

FINAL WORDS FOR PREGNANT WOMEN WITH SCOLIOSIS

Women with scoliosis have nothing to fear when it comes to pregnancy. The changes that happen during pregnancy inside your body are the same that take place with any other women. The only extra care that you need to take is that you need to be careful about your back condition and ensure that you do not overdo things that put an additional pressure on the spine. Follow the guidelines laid by the book so that you can eat right for a healthy spine and a healthy baby. Do the exercises detailed earlier and you should have no cause to worry at all.

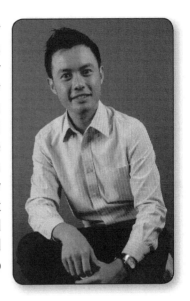

When it comes to pregnancy, you need to be an informed person to be able to wade through the 9 months and after without any significant issues. Assuming that you will have no issues during pregnancy is like having a dream. But then, who does not have issues when it comes to pregnancy. The body goes through so many changes that there are bound to be aspects that you encounter that you have never experienced before.

What you really need to do is read a lot about what is happening in your body and the specific things that you can do in order to ensure that you manage the changes efficiently.

Diet and exercise are the key aspects of managing a pregnancy efficiently. Make sure that the diet that you eat is healthy and conducive to better bone health. And practice the right level of exercise to keep you fighting fit to take the stress when the baby arrives and after.

Women who are strict about their diet and exercise routine experience far lesser issues with the pregnancy and the delivery too.

Remember that there are new researches and techniques that are always coming up to help people face medical conditions and situations better. Keep track of the new researches that are being done to help scoliosis patients deliver more easily.

But one thing is certain that as far as you continue eating right for scoliosis and pregnancy and ensure that you have an active lifestyle, you will be able to sail through your pregnancy and soon hold the new love of your life in your arms.

Take care and best of luck with your baby!

Dr. Kevin Lau D. C.

REFERENCES

1. Warren M.P., Brooks-Gunn J., Hamilton L.H., Warren L.F. and Hamilton W.G. (1986). Scoliosis and fractures in young ballet dancers: relation to delayed menarche and secondary amenorrhea. N Engl J Med, 314:1348—1353.

2. Nowak, A. and Czerwionka-Szaflarska. M. (1998) Clinical picture of mitral valve proplapse syndrome in children - a study of a selfselected material. Med Sci Monit, 4(2): 280-284

3. Akella P., Warren M.P., Jonnavithula S. and Brooks-Gunn J. (Sept, 1991) Scoliosis in ballet dancers. Med Probl Performing Artists. 84—86.

4. Tanchev, P.I., Dzherov, A.D., Parushev, A.D., Dikov, D.M., and Todorov, M.B. (Jun, 2000). Scoliosis in rhythmic gymnasts. Spine, vol 25 (issue 11): 1367-72

5. Omey, M.L., Micheli, L. J. and Gerbino, P.G. (2000). Idiopathic scoliosis and spondylolysis in the female athlete: Tips for treatment. Clinical orthopaedics and related research, 372, 74-84

6. Riseborough E. and Wynne-Davies R. (1973) A genetic survey of idiopathic scoliosis in Boston. J Bone Joint Surg Am, 55:974-982.

7. Czeizel A., Bellyei A., Barta O., et al. (1978) Genetics of adolescent idiopathic scoliosis. J Med Genet, 15:424-427.

8. Weinstein S.L., Zavala D.C. and Ponseti I.V. (Jun, 1981). Idiopathic Scoliosis: long-term follow-up & prognosis in untreated patients. J Bone Joint Surg Am, 63(5): 702-12.

9. Fayssoux, R.S., Cho, R.H. and Herman M.J. (2010) A History of Bracing for Idiopathic Scoliosis in North America Clin Orthop Relat Res, 468:654–64.

10. Coillard C., Circo A.B. and Rivard C.H. (November, 2010) SpineCor treatment for Juvenile Idiopathic Scoliosis: SOSORT award 2010 winner. Scoliosis, 5:25, doi: 10.1186/1748-7161-5-25.

11. Negrini S., Minozzi S., Bettany-Saltikov J., Zaina F., Chockalingam N., Grivas T.B., Kotwicki T., Maruyama T., Romano M. and Vasiliadis E.S. (2010) Braces for idiopathic scoliosis in adolescents. Cochrane Database of Systematic Reviews, Issue 1. Art. No.: CD006850.

12. Dale, E. Rowe, M.D., Saul, M. Bernstein, M.D., Max, F. Riddick, M.D., Adler, F. M.D., Emans. J.B. M.D. and Gardner-Bonneau, D. Ph.D. (May, 1997). A Meta-Analysis of the Efficacy of Non-Operative Treatments for Idiopathic Scoliosis, The Journal of Bone and Joint Surgery 79:664-74.

13. Nachemson, A.L. and Peterson, L.E. (1995). Effectiveness of treatment with a brace in girls who have adolescent idiopathic scoliosis. A prospective, controlled study based on data from the Brace Study of the Scoliosis Research Society. The Journal of Bone and Joint Surgery, 77(6), 815-822.

14. Dolan L.A. and Weinstein SL. (Phila Pa 1976; Sep, 2007) Surgical rates after observation and bracing for adolescent idiopathic scoliosis: an evidence-based review. Spine, 1: 32(19 Suppl): S91-S100.

15. Ogilvie J., Nelson L., Chettier R. and Ward K. (2009) Does bracing alter the natural history of Adolescent Idiopathic Scoliosis? Scoliosis, 4(Suppl 2): O59.

16. Karol L.A. (Phila Pa 1976; Sep, 2001). Effectiveness of bracing in male patients with idiopathic scoliosis, 26(18): 2001-5.

17. Weiss H.R. (Jan 1, 2001). Adolescent Idiopathic Scoliosis: The Effect of Brace Treatment on the Incidence of Surgery. Spine, 26(1), 42-47.

18. Morningstar M.W., Woggon D. and Lawrence G. (Sep, 2004) Scoliosis treatment using a combination of manipulative and rehabilitative therapy: a retrospective case series. BMC Muculoskelet Disord, 14(5): 32. REFERENCES 343

19. Dickson, R. A. and Weinstein, S. L. (Mar, 1999). Bracing (And Screening) — Yes Or No?, British Editorial Society of Bone and Joint Surgery, 81(2): 193-8.

20. Farley, D. (Jul, 1994). Correcting the curved spine of scoliosis - includes related article on X-ray safety. FDA Consumer. 28(6):26-29.

21. Humke T., Grob D., Scheier H. and Siegrist H. (1995) Cotrel-Dubousset and Harrington Instrumentation in idiopathic scoliosis: a comparison of long-term results. Eur Spine J, 4(5): 280-3.

22. Mohaideen A., Nagarkatti D., Banta J.V. and Foley C.L. (Feb, 2007) Not all rods are Harrington - an overview of spinal instrumentation in scoliosis treatment. Pediatr Radiol, 30(2): 110-8.

23. Steinmetz M.P., Rajpal S. and Trost G. (Sep, 2008) Segmental spinal instrumentation in the management of scoliosis. Neurosurgery, 63(3 Suppl): 131-8.

24. Margulies J.Y., Neuwirth M.G., Puri R., Farcy F.V. and MirovskyY. (Apr, 1995) Cotrel Dubousset and Wisconsin segmental spine instrumentation: comparison of results in adolescents with idiopathic scoliosis King Type II. Contemp Orthop, 30(4): 311-4.

25. Sucato D.J. (Phila Pa 1976; Dec, 2010) Management of severe spinal deformity: scoliosis and kyphosis. Spine, 35(25): 2186-92.

26. Shamji M.F. and Isaacs R.E. (Sep, 2008) Anterior-only approaches to scoliosis. Neurosurgery, 63(3 Suppl): 139-48.

27. Wilk B., Karol L.A., Johnston C.E., 2nd, Colby S. and Haideri N. (2006) The Effect of Scoliosis Fusion Surgery on Spinal Ranges of Motion: a Comparison of Fused & Nonfused Patients with

28. Idiopathic Scoliosis. Spine, 31(3): 309-314. 344 HEALTH IN YOUR HANDS

29. Yawn, B.P., Yawn, R.A., Roy A. (Sep 15, 2000). The estimated cost of school scoliosis screening. Spine, 25(18):2387-91.

30. Danielsson, A.J., Wiklund, I. , Pehrsson, K. and Nachemson, A.L. (Aug, 2001). Health-related quality of life in patients with adolescent idiopathic scoliosis: a matched follow-up at least 20 years after treatment with brace or surgery. European Spine Journal. 10(4), 278-288

31. Akazawa1, T., Minami1, S., Takahashi1 K., Kotani1 T., Hanawa T. and Moriya1 H. (Mar, 2005) Corrosion of spinal implants retrieved from patients with scoliosis. J Orthop Sci, 10(2):200-5.

32. Wilk B., MS; Karol L.A., MD; Johnston C.E., II MD; Colby S. and Haideri, N. PhD (Feb 22, 2006). The Effect of Scoliosis Fusion Surgery on Spinal Ranges of Motion: a Comparison of Fused & Nonfused Patients with Idiopathic Scoliosis. Spine, 31(3):309-314.

33. Donovan P. (Mar 21, 2008). Grow Your Own Probiotics, Part 1: Kefir, NaturalNews, Naturalnews.com, http://www.naturalnews. com/022822. html.

34. Nachemson AL, Peterson LE. Effectiveness of treatment with a brace in girls who have adolescent idiopathic scoliosis. A prospective, controlled study based on data from the Brace Study of the Scoliosis Research Society. J Bone Joint Surg Am. June 1995;77(6):815-822.

35. Mary G. Enig, PhD. (Dec 31, 2000). Fatty Acid Requirements for Women, Weston A. Price, wwwwestonaprice.org , http://wwwwestonaprice.org/know-your-fats/fatty-acid-requirements-for-women.

36. Pam Schoenfeld . (Apr 1, 2011). Vitamin B6, The Under-Appreciated Vitamin, Weston A. Price, http://www.westonaprice.org/vitamins-and-minerals/vitamin-b6-the-under-appreciated-vitamin.

37. NRC (National Research Council). Recommended dietary allowances. 10th ed. Washington, DC: National Academy of Sciences, 1989.

38. Clapp JF III. Exercise in pregnancy: a brief clinical review. Fetal Medical Review1990;161:1464–9.

39. Artal R, Wiswell RA, Drinkwater BL, eds. Exercise in pregnancy. 2nd ed. Baltimore: Williams and Wilkins, 1991.

40. Frequently Asked Questions, National Scoliosis Foundation, http://www.scoliosis.org/faq.php.

41. Dr. Stuart Weinstein, Prof of Orthopedic Surgery, University of Iowa. (July, 2008). Scoliosis, Questions and Answers about Scoliosis in Children and, National Institute of Arthiritis and Musculoskeletal and Skin Diseases (NIAMS), http://www.niams.nih.gov/Health_Info/Scoliosis/.

42. Jason C. Eck, DO, MS. Scoliosis, MedicineNet, http://www.medicinenet.com/scoliosis/article.htm.

43. Caroline Arbanas. (Sep 5, 2007). Scoliosis gene discovered, may assist in diagnosis, treatment, Washington University in St. Louis, http://news.wustl.edu/news/Pages/9935.aspx.

44. Raynham, MA. (December 1, 2010). New Study Shows DNA Test Highly Accurate In Predicting Curve Progression in Scoliosis Patients, J&J, http://wwwjnj.com/connect/news/all/new-study-shows-dna-test-highly-accurate-in-predicting-curve-progression-in-scoliosis-patients.

45. Dr. Kevin Lau D.C. (2010), Your Plan for Natural Scoliosis Prevention and Treatment, Health in Your Hands, Third Edition, Pg 33

46. Betz-RR; Bunnell-WP; Lambrecht-Mulier-E; MacEwen-GD J-Bone-Joint-Surg-Am. 1987 Jan; 69(1): 90-6 http://www.scoliosisnutty.com/pregnancy-scoliosis.php.

47. In-Depth Report, Scoliosis, Surgery (November 28, 2011), NY Times, http://health.nytimes.com/health/guides/disease/scoliosis/surgery.html.

48. Singer, Katie, The Garden of Fertility: A Guide to Charting Your Fertility Signals to Prevent or Achieve Pregnancy--Naturally--and to Gauge Reproductive Health, Avery/Penguin, 2004.

49. Built in Birth Control: How Too Much – Or Too Little – Body Fat Could Be Harming Your Fertility, A Special Report from Getting-Pregnant.com, http://www.getting-pregnant.com.

50. Linda Bradley, Menstrual Dysfunction, Cleveland Clinic, Center for Continuing Education, Disease Management Project, http://www.clevelandclinicmeded.com/medicalpubs/diseasemanagement/womens-health/menstrual-dysfunction/.

51. Kristen Burgess. A 7 Part Natural Fertility Course, Getting-Pregnant, http://www.getting-pregnant.com.

52. Lisa Bianco-Davis. (September 20, 2005), Modern Baby Books: Full of Bad Advice Weston A. Price Foundation, http://www.westonaprice.org/childrens-health/modern-baby-books.

53. Guidelines of the American College of Obstetricians and Gynecologists for exercise during pregnancy and the postpartum period, British Journal of Sports Medicine, http://bjsm.bmj.com/cgi/content/full/37/1/6.

54. Weston A. Price Foundation. (January 10, 2004), Diet for Pregnant and Nursing Mothers, Weston A. Price Foundation, http://www.westonaprice.org/childrens-health/diet-for-pregnant-and-nursing-mothers.

55. What to Expect When You're Expecting by Arlene Eisenberg, Heidi E Murkoff & Sandee E Hathaway, BSN, Workman Publishing Company, 2002.

56. Dr. Kevin Lau D.C. (2010), Your Plan for Natural Scoliosis Prevention and Treatment, Health in Your Hands, Third Edition, Pg 77.

57. Sally Fallon and Mary G. Enig, PhD. (March 29, 2002), Vitamin A Saga, Weston A. Price Foundation, http://www.westonaprice.org/fat-soluble-activators/vitamin-a-saga.

58. Jane E. Brody. (October 7. 1995), Study Links Excess Vitamin A and Birth Defects, The New York Times, http://www.nytimes.com/1995/10/07/us/study-links-excess-vitamin-a-and-birth-defects.html.

59. Kenneth J. Rothman and et al. (November 1995), The New England Journal of Medicine: Teratogenicity of High Vitamin A Intake.

60. AAP News Room. (October 13.2008), New Guidelines Double The Amount Of Recommended Vitamin D, American Academy of Pediatrics, http://www.aap.org/pressroom/nce/nce08vitamind.htm.

61. Devereux G. Early life events in asthma – diet. Pediatr Pulmonol. 2007;42(8):663-73.

62. Hoogenboezem, T. Degenhart, H. J. De Muinck Keizer-Schrama, et al., "Vitamin D Metabolism in Breast-Fed Infants and their Mothers," Pediatric Research, 1989; 25: 623-628.

63. Ala-Houhala, M. Koskinen, T. Terho, A. Koivula, T. Visakorpi, J. "Maternal compared with infant vitamin D supplementation," Archives of Disease in Childhood, 1986; 61: 1159-1163.

64. American Academy of Pediatrics, Committee on Nutrition. "The prophylactic requirement and the toxicity of vitamin D," Pediatrics, March 1963; 512-525.

65. Standing Committee on the Scientific Evaluation of Dietary Reference Intakes and its Panel on Folate, Other B Vitamins, and Choline and Subcommittee on Upper Reference Levels of Nutrients, Food and Nutrition Board, Institute of Medicine. Dietary Reference Intakes for Thiamin, Riboflavin, Niacin, Vitamin B6, Folate, Vitamin B12, Pantothenic Acid, Biotin, and Choline. Washington, DC: National Academy Press (1998) pp. 196-305.

66. Kelly P, McPartlin J, Goggins M, Weir DG, Scott JM. Am J Clin Nutr. 1997;65(6):1790-5.

67. Zeisel, SH. The fetal origins of memory: the role of dietary choline in optimal brain development. J Pediatr. 2006;149:S131-S136.

68. Standing Committee on the Scientific Evaluation of Dietary Reference Intakes and its Panel on Folate, Other B Vitamins, and Choline and Subcommittee on Upper Reference Levels of Nutrients, Food and Nutrition Board, Institute of Medicine. Dietary Reference Intakes for Thiamin, Riboflavin, Niacin, Vitamin B6, Folate, Vitamin B12, Pantothenic Acid, Biotin, and Choline. Washington, DC: National Academy Press (1998) pp. 399-422.

69. Rees WD, Wilson FA, Maloney CA. Sulfur amino acid metabolism in pregnancy: the impact of methionine in the maternal diet. J Nutr. 2006;136(6 Suppl):1701S-1705S.

70. Brooks AA, Johnson MR< Steer PJ, Pawson ME, Abdalla HI. Birth weight: nature or nurture? Early Human Dev. 1995;42(1):29-35.

71. Crawford MA. Postgrad Med J 1980 Aug;56(658):557-62.

72. Al MD, van Houwelingen AC, Hornstra G. Am J Clin Nutr 2000 Jan;71(1 Suppl):285S-91S.

73. Dr. Kevin Lau D.C. (2010), Your Plan for Natural Scoliosis Prevention and Treatment, Health in Your Hands, Third Edition, Pg 126.

74. Dr. Kevin Lau D.C. (2010), Your Plan for Natural Scoliosis Prevention and Treatment, Health in Your Hands, Third Edition, Pg 145.

75. Dr. Kevin Lau D.C. (2010), Your Plan for Natural Scoliosis Prevention and Treatment, Health in Your Hands, Third Edition, Pg 180.

76. Dr. Kevin Lau D.C. (2010), Your Plan for Natural Scoliosis Prevention and Treatment, Health in Your Hands, Third Edition, Pg 89.

INDEX

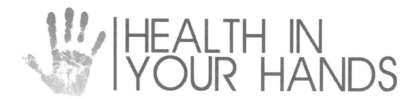

HEALTH IN YOUR HANDS

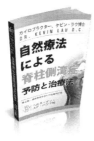 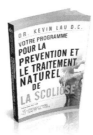 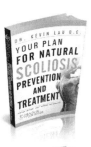

A completely natural, safe, tried and tested diet and exercise program to treat and prevent scoliosis!

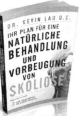 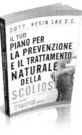 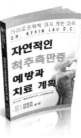

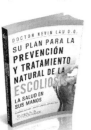 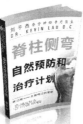 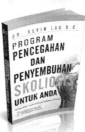

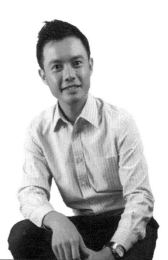

In "Your Plan for Natural Scoliosis Prevention and Correction" you will:

- Uncover the most recent research on the true causes of scoliosis.
- Discover how bracing and surgery treat merely the symptom not the root cause of scoliosis.
- Find out what latest treatment work, what doesn't and why.
- The most common symptoms scoliosis sufferers have.
- How a quick scoliosis assessment of a teenager can help with their quality of life in later years.
- The only book in the world that treats scoliosis by controlling how scoliosis genes are expressed.
- In-depth understanding of how muscles and ligaments work on the common types of scoliosis.
- Customize an exercise routine unique to your scoliosis to suit even the busiest schedule.
- What are the most effective exercises for scoliosis and what should be avoided at all cost.
- Tips and tricks to modify your posture and body mechanics to decrease scolisosis back pain.
- The best sitting, standing and sleeping postures for scoliosis.
- Learn from others with scoliosis in inspirational stories and case studies.

ScolioTrack

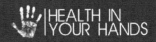

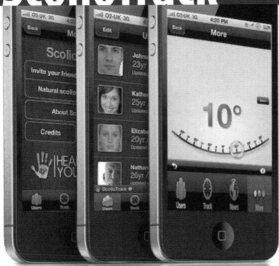

Scoliotrack is a safe and innovative way to track a person's scoliosis condition month to month by using the iPhone accelerometer just as a doctor would with a scoliometer. A scoliometer is an instrument that is used to estimate the amount of curve in a person's spine. It may be used as a tool during screening or as follow-up for scoliosis, a deformity in which the spine curves abnormally.

Features of program

- Can be used with multiple users and saves their data conveniently on the iphone for future checkups

- Tracks and saves a person's Angle of Trunk Rotation (ATR), a key measurement in screening for and planning treatment of scoliosis.

- Tracks a person's height and weight – ideal for growing teenagers with scoliosis or adults who are health conscious.

- Scoliosis progression is graphed making it easy to read month to month changes to a persons scoliosis.

- Displays the latest news feed for scoliosis to keep users informed and up-to-date.

- Full help and easy to follow guides so anyone can track their scoliosis in the comfort of their own home

---

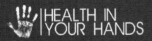

Exercise DVD

Broken down into three easy-to-digest sections, the DVD will take you through the various steps in order to start rebuilding and re-balancing your spine. The comprehensive sections cover everything from Body Balancing Stretches to Building Your Core and a number of different Body Alignment Exercises that have all been carefully designed and selected by Dr Kevin Lau.

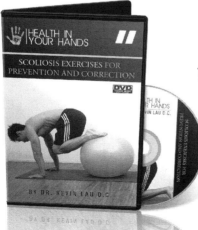

The advantages of the DVD are:

- It gives a 60-minute concise expansion of Dr Lau's book by the same name,
- Health In Your Hands: Your Plan for Natural Scoliosis Prevention and Treatment.
- The Body Balancing section in the DVD explains in detail the correct stretching techniques for scoliosis sufferers to relieve stiffness.
- The Building Your Core section focuses on strengthening the muscles that give stability to your spine.
- Body Alignment Exercises will improve the overall alignment of your spine.
- All the exercises that feature in the DVD are suitable for pre and post-operative rehabilitation for scoliosis conditions.

STAY CONNECTED

Stay connected with the latest health tips, news and updates from Dr. Lau with the following social media sites. Join the Health In Your Hands page on Facebook to have the opportunity to ask Dr. Kevin Lau questions about the book, general questions about their scoliosis, iPhone App called ScolioTrack or the exercise DVD:

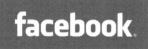

www.facebook.com/HealthInYourHands

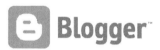

www.DrKevinLau.blogspot.com

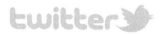

www.twitter.com/DrKevinLau

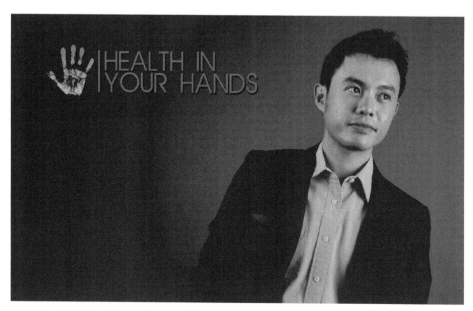

Made in the USA
San Bernardino, CA
19 March 2013